Hypertension

And

Rational Design of Captopril, the First ACE Inhibitor for the Treatment of Hypertension

By

Hong Son Cheung

Kabel Publishers

* 1998 *

KABEL PUBLISHERS
ISBN 1-57529-094-4
11225 Huntover Drive
Rockville, MD 20852-3613
Phone/Fax (301)468-64634 * (301)2312-3613
E-Mail:KABELCOMP@EROLS.COM

To

my mother Lee Tsing Chin

To

my two sons Noland and Alvin Cheung

Acknowledgements

The author would like to thank those who supported his works in writing this book in every event. In alphabetical order they were Alvin Cheung, Anna Tang, Chia-Ching Chao, Charles Dorso, Helen Lee, Lynn Roger, Lisa and Noland Cheung, Reena Cheung and RoseAnn Baska.

The author also would like to thank those who revised this book with all kind suggestions. They were Alvin Cheung, Charles Dorso, Lisa and Noland Cheung, Ken Dickson and Shih-Jung Lan.

Contents

Introduction

Hypertension is a common disease in humans. The causes of hypertension are more clear today. Although treatment of hypertension is well controlled by certain drugs, there are still a lot of unanswered questions. The purpose of this article is to relate the cause of hypertension with drug treatment. The design of the first ACE inhibitor, CAPOTEN® or Captopril (an anti-hypertensive drug), is also presented here. In addition, some other thoughts for making drugs are also included.

CAPOTEN® is a registered trademark of Bristol-Myers Squibb Inc.

Chapter I

Blood pressure measurements

Normal blood pressure, systolic and diastolic pressure

The measurement of blood pressure generates two values, one high and the other low, such as 125/75. The high value (125) is referred to as systolic pressure, and the low value (75) is referred to as diastolic pressure. The range considered as normal blood pressure is between 115 to 128 for the systolic measurement and between 72 to 85 for the diastolic measurement. Patients with values below or above either range were considered as either hypotensive or hypertensive, respectively. Large populations of patients were found to be hypertensive. The following discussion is focused on the heart to lower blood pressure of the hypertensive patient.

Brief history of blood pressure measurement

4000 years ago, the yellow emperor of China, Huang-Ti, was aware of the importance of the changing characteristics of the pulse. With remarkable prescience, he commented that people who ate too much salt had hard pulses and tended to suffer strokes (O'Brien and Fitzgerald, 1994).

Every day, all over the world, many thousands of physicians, nurses and paramedics measure systemic arterial pressure by applying a cuff with an inflatable bladder around the patients' arms and using a stethoscope to listen to the sounds in the brachial artery. Many care providers know that they are listening to "Korotkoff sounds," but very few are aware that the method was introduced 90 years ago by a Russian doctor and scientist named Nikolai Sergeevich Korotkoff (Shevchenko and Tsitlik, 1996). Thus, blood pressure could be measured with the application of an elastic, rubber cuff of the Riva-Rocci apparatus: pressure in the cuff is increased until the blood supply to the periphery is completely stopped. Then, the pressure in the cuff was decreased and a stethoscope was used to listen to the pressure in the artery "directly below the cuff." Once the pressure fell below a certain level, the first short tones could be heard; this indicated the passage of the first pulse wave along the artery below the cuff. The manometer reading at which the first tone appeared corresponded to the systolic pressure. With a further decrease in pressure in the cuff, tones were replaced by murmurs that were followed, in turn, by second tones. Finally, all the sounds disappeared. The moment all sounds subsided, according to Korotkoff, led to the conclusion that blood was flowing freely through the arteries. The diastolic pressure in the artery at that moment slightly exceeded the pressure in the cuff, and the manometer reading, at the moment that the sounds disappeared, corresponded to the diastolic pressure (Shevchenko and Tsitlik, 1996).

Korotkoff considered the tones and murmurs in the vessel to be compression sounds. He thought the tones were caused by the rushing "of a minuscule part of the pulse wave" through the compressed area during a very short interval. Also, vibration of the "unsticking" vessel walls contributed to the production of the tones. Korotkoff believed that the sound phenomenon depended on the elastic properties of the arterial walls (Shevchenko and Tsitlik, 1996). This explanation is quite correct. However, it is still not clear why the tones completely disappeared when the blood was flowing freely through the arteries after the last tone. Why can't the pulse be detected even while using the stethoscope in the absence of external pressure applied with the aid of the cuff? The mechanism used to detect the pulse signal is not explained at all by the measuring instrument.

Heart pressure

The function of the heart only contributes two (2) different blood pressures. One is from the heart pumping and driving out the blood from the heart to the artery during the heart's contraction. This pressure is referred to as theoretical systolic pressure, (maximum pressure applied from the heart) giving the pressure with the higher value. The other pressure is the blood completely returning back and filling the heart during its relaxation.

This blood pressure is the control pressure of the heart. It is referred to as theoretical diastolic pressure (minimum blood pressure in heart, control, background and reference pressure) and is the blood pressure of lower value.

Mechanism of blood pressure measurement

The blood pressure believes to be "measured" that is measuring the blood pressure, but, in fact it is not true and correctly it is detecting the presence of

12

the pulse. This pulse is detected in the arm artery from the heart's beat in the cycle of contraction and relaxation of the heart. The pulse can only be heard with the aid of a stethoscope in the presence of external pressure applied using a cuff wrapped around the arm. There is a range of the application of the external pressure in which the pulse can be detected. The applied external pressure must be in the range between the highest pressure (systolic pressure) and lowest pressure (diastolic pressure) from the heart. If the external pressure is higher than the systolic pressure, no pulse can be heard because the artery cannot be moved (vibrated) in the measured position.

Mechanically, the pulse can be heard or detected (signal picked up) because the pulse wave is formed. The pulse wave occurs from heart pressures of contraction and relaxation in one single cycle. Contraction produces high pressure. Relaxation produces low pressure. The pressures of the heart generate a pattern (direction) of the high pressure and then low pressure in one single cycle (or low pressure and then high pressure). The next cycle is also showing the same pressure pattern (direction): again high and then low (or low and then high). Thus, the pulse wave can be formed. This pulse wave is then converted to a sound. However, the sound in this case is too weak to detect even using the stethoscope.

For the purpose of detecting the pulse, a booster (amplifier) is required. The cuff which generates the external pressure is the booster. This booster uses three different pressures to achieve the goal of recreating the above pressure pattern and a detectable sound. In these three pressures, one of the pressures is external pressure applied around the arm. The stethoscope must be in the position near the booster (external pressure) around the arm and at the location of the artery. The other two pressures are natural pressures of the heart's highest (systolic pressure) and lowest pressure (diastolic pressure). The external pressure is in the range between the heart's two pressures.

The external pressure is lower than the systolic pressure but higher than the diastolic pressure. This external pressure alternates against the higher systolic and then lower diastolic pressure in one single cycle. The middle (in this case, lower) external pressure against the higher systolic pressure around the arm produces the condition (direction) of high pressure. It is also the middle (in this case, higher) external pressure against the lower diastolic pressure around the arm that produces the condition (direction) of low pressure. The pattern of pressures of high and then low (or low then high) occurs. Accordingly the pulse wave is formed. As a result, the pulse can be detected in this case.

If the external pressure is higher than the systolic pressure, it is certainly higher than the diastolic pressure as well. It is also true that if the external pressure is lower than the diastolic pressure then it is certainly lower than the systolic pressure. The higher external pressure alternates against both lower systolic and lower diastolic pressures in one single cycle around the arm. This situation produces both conditions (directions) of low pressures. The lower external pressure against the higher diastolic pressure and certainly higher systolic pressure produces both conditions (directions) of high pressures. The pattern of high pressure and then low pressure cannot be obtained in these 2 cases. Thus, the pulse wave cannot occur and the pulse certainly cannot be detected.

For these reasons, during the detection of the pulse, begin with the external pressure which is higher than the systolic pressure. It is also higher than the diastolic pressure. In this case, the pattern of high and then low pressure does not occur. The pulse, thus, cannot be detected. The external pressure is gradually reduced to just lower than the systolic pressure. The external pressure, of course, is higher than the diastolic pressure. Now the external pressure is between the systolic and diastolic pressure. As mentioned above, the pattern of high and then low is completed. As a result, the pulse wave is formed. The pulse, therefore, can be detected. Until the external pressure gradually drops to just below the diastolic pressure, then the external pressure is lower than both diastolic and systolic pressure. The high and low pattern cannot occur again. The pulse, therefore, cannot be detected and "disappears".

During pulse detection, the first pulse can be heard only when the applied external pressure gradually drops just below the highest heart pressure. The completed pulse cycle is beginning. The applied external pressure reading at this first detected pulse is the blood pressure and is referred to as true systolic pressure. And the last pulse can be heard only when the external pressure has dropped to a level just above the lowest heart pressure. Below the lowest heart pressure, the pulse cycle cannot be completed anymore. The applied external pressure reading for the last detected pulse is the blood pressure and is referred to as true diastolic pressure. As mentioned above, the external pressure readings for the first and last pulse are just a little below or above the highest and lowest pressures performed by the heart, respectively. The difference between these true pressure readings and theoretical pressures of systolic and diastolic from the heart is almost insignificant. Thus, these readings may be considered as theoretical and true systolic and diastolic pressures.

During the measurement of the blood pressure, the first pulse that can be heard, is extremely weak and then becomes louder than the previous pulse. The first pulse can be heard, as mentioned above, only in the condition where the applied external pressure has gradually dropped just below the highest heart pressure (systolic pressure). The difference between the highest heart pressure and the applied external pressure in this case is almost insignificant. The amplitude of the first detected formed pulse wave therefore, is very small and is thus, converted to a weak sound. Each pulse obtained follows the previous pulse. The difference now between the highest heart pressure (fixed pressure) and the gradually decreased applied external pressure (pressure always changed) becomes larger and larger until reaching a maximum. The amplitude of the pulse wave formed from each pulse after another is larger and larger. The detected pulse heard, therefore, becomes louder and louder until reaching a maximum. At the end, the pulse can be heard weak again and then, suddenly has completely disappeared after the last pulse.

Relationship of systolic and diastolic pressure

Systolic pressure (pumping pressure, high value) and diastolic pressure (control pressure, low value) are related and influenced by each other to some degree. The major influence for systolic and diastolic pressure is not really from each other. This will be explained as follows based on a hypothetical concept.

It has been found that in some patients treated with an ACE inhibitor [ACE inhibitor blocks angiotensin II (AII) formation from the activity of Angiotensin-converting enzyme (ACE)], anthypertensive agent, the systolic pressure was lowered significantly but not the diastolic pressure. Using drugs of β-blocker or calcium channel blocker classes to treat these hypertensive patients, blood pressure dropped because the heart rate was reduced (calcium channel blocker decreases contractility of heart). However, these patients usually showed a similar blood pressure decrease by treatment with any of the above drugs. The systolic pressure was much easier to reduce but not the diastolic pressure. For these patients, treatment with the above mentioned drugs decreased both the systolic and the diastolic pressure significantly, but the diastolic was still high. It was hard to drop the pressure any further especially for the diastolic pressure. Even a diuretic agent added to the above drugs could control pressure in some patients, but not all. Diastolic pressure was the more difficult to lower. Systolic pressure was much easier to lower.

Hypertension, systolic pressure and vasoconstriction

The systolic pressure is the pressure achieved when the blood is pumped out by the heart and driven to the artery (highest pressure from the heart). If there is a resistance to the flowing of the blood, the systolic pressure is elevated. In vasoconstriction of blood vessels, the diameter of the vessel becomes narrow and the resistance to blood flowing in the vessel is increased. The systolic pressure is, of course, elevated. This condition will influence the diastolic pressure slightly but not greatly. The higher systolic pressure may suggest that vasoconstriction plays most of the role possibly from Angiotensin II (AII) formation (explained in Chapters 2 and 3). AII is a vasoconstrictor well known to cause hypertension. ACE inhibitors can abolish the AII formation and lower the systolic pressure in hypertensive patients greatly (explained in Chapter 3). However, it is not nearly as great for diastolic pressure. This is also the situation found in those patients.

Hypertension, diastolic pressure and total volume of blood in the heart

The diastolic pressure is the pressure of the blood that is completely returning and filling the heart. The total volume of the blood exerts a pressure in the heart. This pressure is the diastolic pressure. This pressure is a control pressure of heart (reference pressure, lowest pressure from the heart). The diastolic pressure is controlled directly by the total volume of blood in the heart. Therefore, the resistance is not influenced significantly.

For example, when blowing air into a balloon, there is a pressure in the balloon. The balloon pressure depends on how much air was blown in. The total amount of air in the balloon controls the extent of the pressure. This pressure is similar to the diastolic pressure that results from the total volume of blood in the heart. Thus, the diastolic pressure depends on the total amount (total volume) of blood in the heart. Without reducing the total volume of blood in the heart, the pressure exerted in heart will stay the same (control pressure from total volume of blood in heart). The total volume of blood in the heart, if reduced, will reduce the pressure automatically. There is no way to remove blood from the system for treatment of the patients.

A large portion of blood is water. Water can be removed instead of blood in the system, thus, to lower the total volume of blood in heart. The diastolic pressure, therefore, can be reduced. The higher diastolic pressure, thus, is considered likely from more volume of blood in the heart than the normal total volume. This proposal can explain why diastolic pressure is more difficult to lower by drug treatment with ACE inhibitor, β-blocker or Calcium channel blocker.

Low blood pressure

Low blood pressure in patients can also be explained in this fashion. The total volume of blood in the heart is lower than the corrected total volume of blood in the heart. Increasing the total volume of blood in heart is the way for the treatment of the patients having low blood pressure.

Personal evidence

This is just a theory, a concept. Combining all the proposals in this book, I have tried them collectively on myself as a guinea pig under the observation of a physician.* My high blood pressure was the same as some other hypertensive patients. The diastolic pressure, especially, was not well controlled for more than 10 years with various treatments. Recently my blood pressure surprisingly dropped from a high to low blood pressure (92/72) after three weeks of food intake totally without a minimal amount of salt along with the ACE inhibitor, angiotensin II receptor antagonist and diuretic agent treatment. Afterwards, eating the right amount of sodium salt in the food would increase the water level in the body. My blood pressure was found later to be changed to normal (115-125/75-82).

In conclusion blood pressure measurement has been known for 100 years. Knowledge of using instruments to measure blood pressure is well established. However, understanding the mechanism of the function for blood pressure measuring is still not entirely clear. The following is based on scientific experience, a hypothetical concept, common sense and a mechanistic point of view.

(1) Higher systolic pressure is possibly due to AII mediated vaso-constriction.

(2) Higher diastolic pressure is possibly due to more total volume of blood in heart.

(3) The patients with low blood pressure may have an inadequate total volume of blood in the heart.

The mechanism of the measurement of the blood pressure at the measured position is detecting the presence of the pulse from the cycle of contraction and relaxation of the heart. It actually is not measuring blood pressure. This pulse (complete pulse wave or beat) can be detected at the position of the arm on which the external pressure is applied. The continuous external pressure must alternate with being against the highest and then the lowest pressure from the heart (systolic and diastolic, respectively). External pressure must be between these two different pressures from the heart. The pulse wave from the pattern of high pressure and then low pressure can be formed and therefore, the pulse can be detected. If the external pressure is higher or lower than the systolic or diastolic pressure, then the external pressure alternates with being either against two low pressures of systolic and diastolic or two high pressures of systolic and diastolic. Thus, the pattern of the high pressure and then low pressure cannot be completed. The pulse wave is not formed and, thus, no pulse can be detected.

Chapter II

Hypertension

Angiotensin-converting enzyme (ACE) plays a very important role in this disease (Skeggs et al., 1956). Angiotensin II (AII) is a potent vasoconstrictor identified as an etiological factor in the pathogenesis of some forms of hypertensive disease. It is derived from the catalytic reaction of the enzyme ACE from the naturally occurring substrate Angiotensin I (AI) (Skeggs et al., 1954; Skeggs et al., 1956) in the renin-angiotensin system (Fig. 1).

Bradykinin is a nonapeptide product of kallikrein. It is a vasodilator which causes a hypotensive effect. The same enzyme ACE also cleaves bradykinin to its products (Yang et al., 1970; Erdös, 1977; Cheung, 1996) and thus, this hypotensive effect is lost (Fig. 1).

AII can be further cleaved by aminopeptidase (angiotensinase) to Angiotensin III (AIII) (Blair-West et al., 1971; Cambell et al., 1974; Goodfriend and Peach, 1975). AIII is found to stimulate aldosterone release. Aldosterone will have sodium ion retaining ability. Sodium salt has strong ability to absorb water. Thus, the sodium ion retention also causes water retention (Fig. 1).

By blocking the enzymatic action of ACE using inhibitor drugs, such as captopril (Cushman and Ondetti, 1980; Cheung, 1996), AII and AIII formation and bradykinin degradation would be prevented (Figs. 1 and 2). Thus, blood pressure would be lowered in many hypertensive patients.

A. Vasoconstriction

One of the major causes for the hypertension is vasoconstriction. AII is a truly potent vasoconstrictor formed from its substrate AI by the enzymatic cleavage action of ACE. Using an ACE inhibitor such as captopril blocks the formation of AII. The vasoconstriction effect is therefore also blocked (Fig. 1).

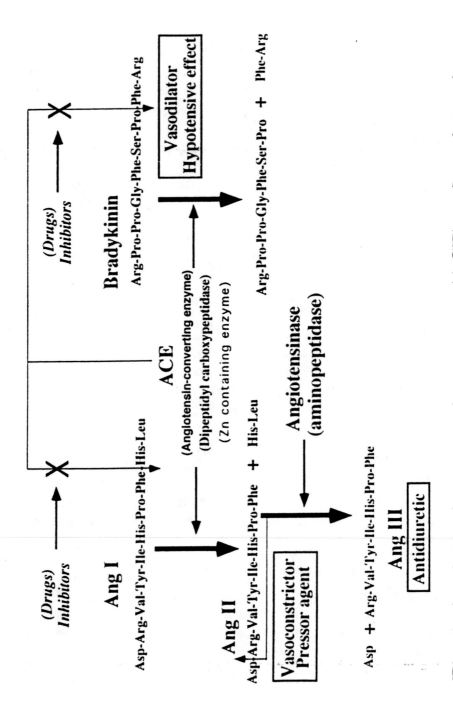

Fig. 1. Angiotensin-converting enzyme (ACE) and angiotensinase

Angiotensin II and angiotensin II receptor

Elevating blood pressure requires both AII and AII receptors bound together (Chiu et al. 1988; Wong et al. 1989; Chiu et al. 1990). After binding, vasoconstriction results. The AII receptor antagonist such as Cozaar® (registered trademark of Merck & Co., Inc.) can block the binding between AII and AII receptors. Thus, high blood pressure resulting from vasoconstriction is lowered (Fig. 2).

ACE inhibitor and Angiotensin II receptor antagonist

Both the ACE inhibitor and AII receptor antagonist are focused on AII, to lower blood pressure by inhibiting the AII formation from ACE action and by blocking the binding between AII and AII receptor, respectively. Both are very effective and potent drugs for treating hypertension mediated by vasoconstriction.

Bradykinin and AII receptor antagonist

ACE inhibitors not only block AII formation, but also bradykinin degradation (Cheung, 1996). In this case, blood pressure is lowered, but, coughing and itching occur in some patients because bradykinin is present. It is a naturally occuring factor in the body which causes itching and coughing (Chan et al. 1993; Fletcher. et al. 1994; Lacourciere. et al. 1994). AII receptor antagonist lowers blood pressure by blocking binding of AII and its receptor, but, it does not inhibit the ACE action. Thus, AII formation and bradykinin degradation are maintained and the itching and coughing effect of the bradykinin, therefore, disappear (Fig. 2). Patients who are treated with ACE inhibitor and found to have itching and coughing can switch to AII receptor antagonist to stop this problem. In addition, high blood pressure from vasoconstriction is also under contr∪

ACE inhibitor and Diuretic agent

In some patients treated with ACE inhibitor, blood pressure was lowered initially but rose later. A diuretic agent, such as HCTZ, can be added together with the ACE inhibitor to control their blood pressure. The patients requiring this treatment are classified as low renin hypertensives (Rubin and Antonaccio, 1980) (Fig. 3).

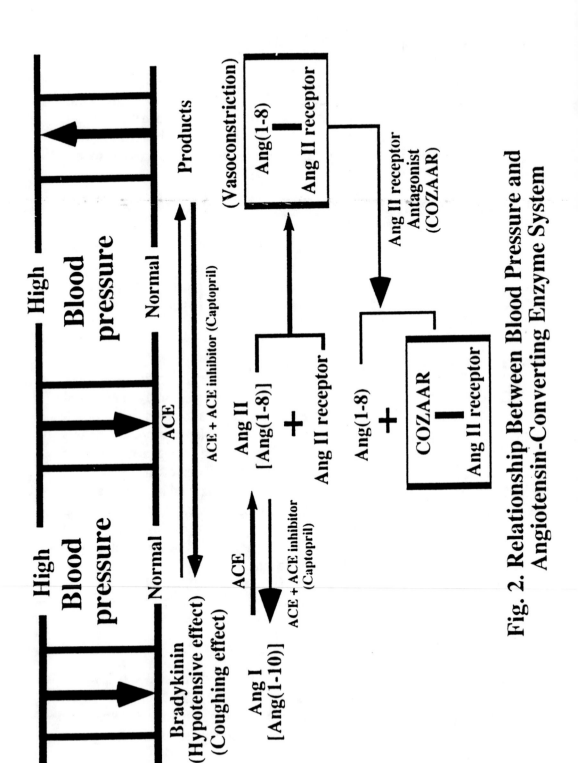

Fig. 2. Relationship Between Blood Pressure and Angiotensin-Converting Enzyme System

22

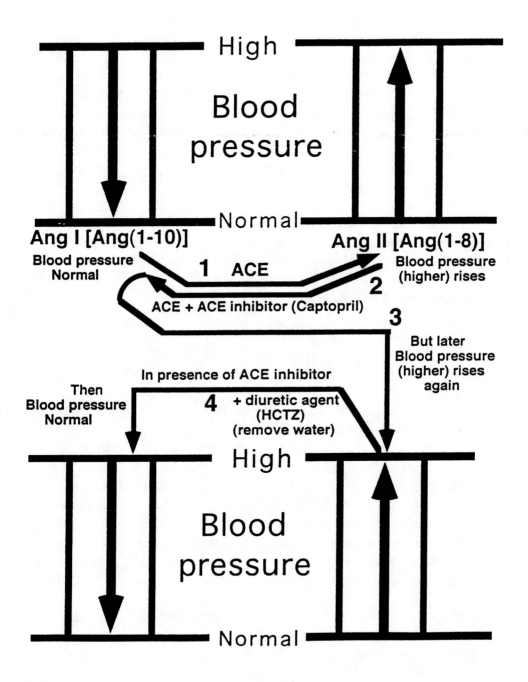

Fig 3. Low Renin Hypertensive Patients

Questions

Several questions remain: (1) Why, in some patients treated with ACE inhibitor, did the blood pressure which was lower in the beginning, rise later? (2) Why was blood pressure controlled, after a diuretic agent was added with the ACE inhibitor? Was it possibly a water retention mechanism that was involved? (3) Why were patients treated with ACE inhibitor and diuretic agent classified as low renin hypertension? (4) Why did low renin hypertensive patient require both ACE inhibitor and diuretic agent treatment?

Explanations and proposals

I carefully reviewed all available published information and combined this with my experience. The above issues, thus, can be well explained. However, this proposal is purely hypothetical without direct experimental proof, but the hypothetical ideas are based all on the experiment of evidence and with the judgment of personal experience.

B. Water retention

Water retention, Angiotensin III, sodium and potassium ion

The second major cause or mechanism of hypertension is water retention. As mentioned above, AII is further cleaved to AIII by aminopeptidase. AIII will cause aldosterone release. Aldosterone results in sodium ion retention. Sodium salt such as sodium chloride has a strong ability to absorb water. Therefore, sodium ion remaining in the body also causes water retention (water remaining in the body). Potassium ion has the same property as sodium ion. Theoretically, potassium ion in the body also will cause water retention and hypertension. However, the amount of potassium ion in the body is much less than sodium ion, at least 30 time less than sodium in the blood. Thus, the potassium ion will not contribute to water retention at all.

An ACE inhibitor blocks AII formation. It is also stopping AIII formation. Water retention from the pathway of AIII cannot occur in the presence of an ACE inhibitor (Figs. 1 and 2).

Blood pressure rises later after ACE inhibitor treatment alone

As mentioned above, in some patients treated with an ACE inhibitor such as captopril by itself, blood pressure was lowered in the beginning. It then rose later (Fig. 3). When the diuretic agent, HCTZ, was added together with an ACE inhibitor, the high blood pressure was again lowered and controlled. Treatment by diuretic agent alone was ineffective.

In the treatment with ACE inhibitor alone, the ACE inhibitor inhibited AII formation from AI by ACE cleavage action (Figs. 1, 2 and 3). Hypertension mediated by AII vasoconstriction and water retention by AIII was completely abolished. The AI concentration built up because of the ACE inhibitor presence (Figs. 1, 2 and 3). The later blood pressure increase must be related to the large amount of AI built up in the presence of ACE inhibitor. There might be another mechanism for hypertension from AI in the renin-angiotensin system besides AII from ACE.

Water retention in renin-angiotensin system: Ang(1-7) and neutral endopeptidase (NEP)

The addition of a diuretic agent to an ACE inhibitor lowered and controlled blood pressure. This strongly suggested that the later rise in blood pressure was probably due to water retention.

From the above information, in the presence of ACE inhibitors, a large amount of AI accumulated and after an additional diuretic agent was used, a large amount of water was removed from the body. This water retention was possibly related to the large amount of AI present. AI, by itself, did not show any effect on water retention. It might be due to a new product of AI cleavage by the action of unknown enzyme. In my judgment and experience, neutral endopeptidase (NEP) was the right candidate for this cleavage action, cleaving AI [Ang(1-10)] directly to Ang(1-7) in the body. The Ang(1-7) was shown to have a potent antidiuretic effect (Santos and Campagnole-Sanyos, 1994).

The Ang(1-7) presence in the body can then lead to the reasonable assumption that it causes the water retention effect. With only ACE in-hibitor treatment in hypertensive patients, the high blood pressure mediated by AII vasoconstriction is blocked. Water retention resulting from the formation of Ang(1-7) by neutral endopeptidase action can occur. The blood pressure, however, will still be high. A diuretic agent, such as HCTZ, is required to be added to the treatment of ACE inhibitor. Blood pressure, thus, can be controlled. As a result, this hypothesis can explain the above mentioned treatment requiring both ACE inhibitor and diuretic agent (Fig. 4).

Water retention and atrial natriuretic peptide or factor

AI is not the only substrate for neutral endopeptidase. Atrial natriuretic peptide or factor (ANP or ANF) is also a naturally occurring substrate for NEP (Fig. 5). ANP showed both natriuretic and diuretic effects (Wilkins, et al., 1993; Seymour, et al., 1994). Natriuretic and diuretic effects mean the removal of sodium and water from the body, respectively. ANP, after the cleavage action by NEP to the product of ring opened ANP, lost the ability of the natriuretic and diuretic effects. The sodium and water cannot be removed and will remain in the body. Water retention can reasonably be assumed to have occurred. ANP degradation is another water retention mechanism for hypertension.

Water retention and neutral endopeptidase (NEP)

Both mechanisms of water retention are derived from the same enzyme activity of NEP on the substrates AI and ANP to the products Ang(1-7) and ring opened ANP, respectively. An inhibitor could be designed to block NEP activity. Theoretically, after inhibition of NEP by its inhibitor, the Ang(1-7) and ring opened ANP cannot be formed. Both mechanisms for water retention by Ang(1-7) and ring opened ANP, therefore, are abolished simultaneously.

NEP inhibitor

Many NEP inhibitors have already been synthesized. SQ 28603 was a potent NEP inhibitor (Delaney et al., 1994). As mentioned above, NEP cleavage of AI to Ang(1-7) was just a proposal, a hypothetical concept. No experiments have been done for this yet. However NEP inhibitor evidence already exists, that by inhibiting the product formation of ring opened ANP formed by NEP activity, more water was excreted in the urine (Wilkins et al. 1993).

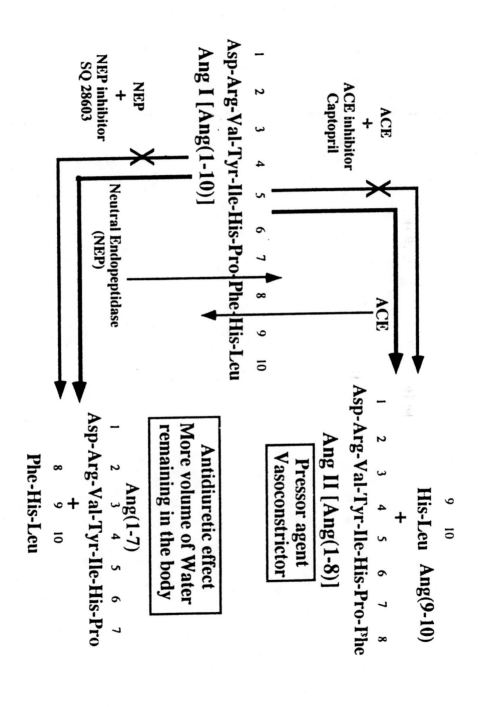

Fig. 4. Proposal from Hypothetical Concept

27

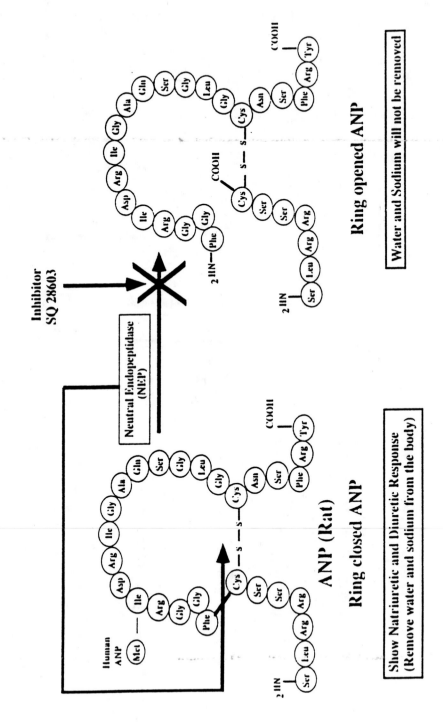

Fig. 5. Activity of Neutral Endopeptidase (NEP)

The evidence clearly showed that NEP inhibitor SQ 28603 inhibited NEP activity, thus, resulting in an anti-water retention effect (natriuretic and diuretic effect) from blocking the degradation of ring closed ANP. There is no evidence to prove that Ang(1-7) was also involved to have this anti-water retention effect from this NEP inhibition. However, if this mechanism of Ang(1-7) is truly present, NEP inhibition is not just blocking the degradation of ANP by NEP action. It will also abolish the formation of Ang(1-7) by NEP action. This water retention from Ang(1-7) could be automatically prevented in this NEP inhibition. Thus, SQ 28603 inhibited NEP activity, not just for the ANP degradation, but possibly also for the formation of Ang(1-7) from the substrate AI. The effect of water retention from Ang(1-7) was, thus, also abolished. Using a diuretic will have the same effect of removing water. This proposal from a hypothetical point of view could explain why in some patients treated with an ACE inhibitor alone, blood pressure dropped in the beginning and later rose. The blood pressure could be under control after a diuretic agent was added together with ACE inhibitor.

This hypothetical proposal explains the above questions (1) and (2). The questions (3) and (4) remain unanswered. Questions (3) and (4) can also be answered by this proposal.

NEP, angiotensin I and angiotensinogen

The hypothetical concept proposed above indicates that another mechanism of hypertension from water retention was involved in the renin-angiotensin system by the enzyme activity of NEP (Fig. 4). NEP is possibly involved in the renin-angiotensin system to cleave the same substrate of ACE, AI. The NEP cleaves the AI molecule at the bond between the amino acids of proline and phenylalanine (Fig. 4 and 6). AI is not the only substrate for NEP. The angiotensinogen (AI precursor) possibly is also a substrate for NEP. It could also be cleaved at exactly the same bond, the same position as in AI structure by NEP directly to the product Ang(1-7) (Fig. 6). There is no evidence to show this action. From experience and the property of the enzyme, it strongly suggests this possibility that the NEP cleaves the substrate of renin, angiotensinogen, directly to the product Ang(1-7). This is another proposal from a hypothetical concept.

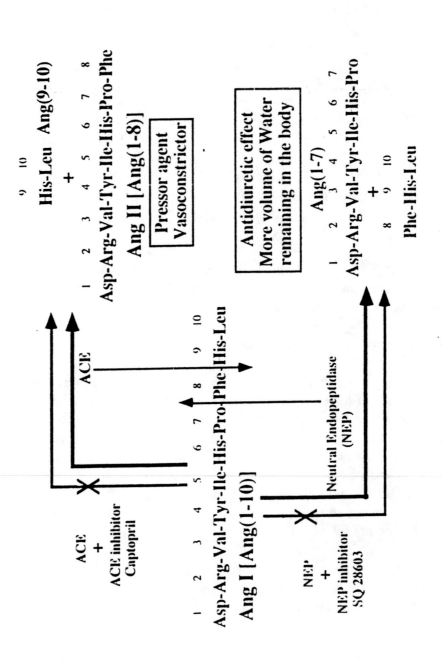

Fig. 4. Proposal from Hypothetical Concept

30

Correction for p. 30, Fig. 6

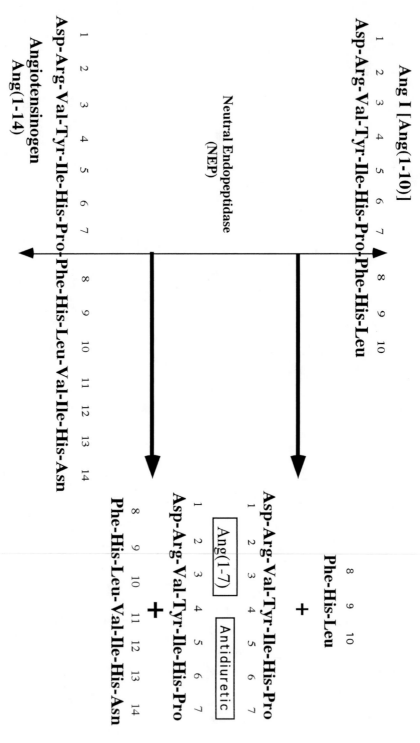

Ang I [Ang(1-10)]

1 2 3 4 5 6 7 8 9 10
Asp-Arg-Val-Tyr-Ile-His-Pro-Phe-His-Leu

Neutral Endopeptidase
(NEP)

8 9 10
Phe-His-Leu

Asp-Arg-Val-Tyr-Ile-His-Pro
1 2 3 4 5 6 7

+

Ang(1-7)   Antidiuretic

Asp-Arg-Val-Tyr-Ile-His-Pro
1 2 3 4 5 6 7

+

8 9 10 11 12 13 14
Phe-His-Leu-Val-Ile-His-Asn

1 2 3 4 5 6 7 8 9 10 11 12 13 14
Asp-Arg-Val-Tyr-Ile-His-Pro-Phe-His-Leu-Val-Ile-His-Asn
Angiotensinogen
Ang(1-14)

Fig. 6. The proposal of Neutral Endopeptidase in Renin-angiotensin system

PRA (Plasma renin activity): measures the amount of Ang I formation from its precursor substrate angiotensinogen by enzyme renin in plasma.

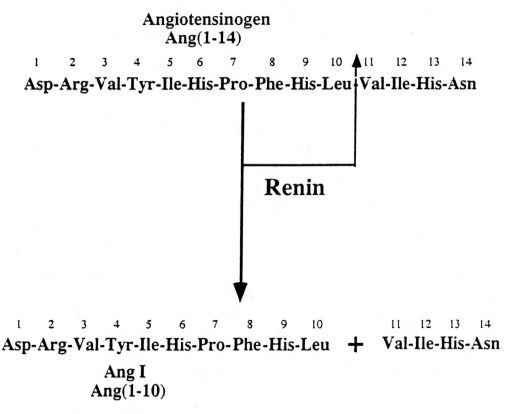

Angiotensinogen
Ang(1-14)

| 1 | 2 | 3 | 4 | 5 | 6 | 7 | 8 | 9 | 10 | 11 | 12 | 13 | 14 |

Asp-Arg-Val-Tyr-Ile-His-Pro-Phe-His-Leu┊Val-Ile-His-Asn

Renin

| 1 | 2 | 3 | 4 | 5 | 6 | 7 | 8 | 9 | 10 | | 11 | 12 | 13 | 14 |

Asp-Arg-Val-Tyr-Ile-His-Pro-Phe-His-Leu + Val-Ile-His-Asn

Ang I
Ang(1-10)

Fig. 7. Renin activity in renin-angiotensin system

31

Low renin (Low PRA)

Patients, treated with ACE inhibitor and diuretic agent together, were found to be low renin hypertensive patients (Fig. 3). Low renin is referred to as low plasma renin activity. Plasma renin activity (PRA) is renin activity measured in plasma (Fig. 7). Pharmacologists considered PRA was related only to the amount of renin (enzyme) present in plasma. In the literature, low renin (low PRA) meant low amount of renin present in plasma.

Renin and/or angiotensinogen ?

Renin is the enzyme, in the renin-angiotensin system which cleaves its substrate angiotensinogen to the product AI. PRA is a measure of the amount of AI formed from angiotensinogen by the cleavage activity of the enzyme renin (Fig. 7). Enzyme activity does not only depend on the amount of enzyme. It also depends on the amount of substrate. Thus, the amount of AI formation (renin activity) depends on both the amounts of the enzyme renin and substrate angiotensinogen used (Figs. 7 and 8). In the low renin patients, low renin results obtained in this case should not be referred to as low amount of renin. It should really be referred to as low amount of substrate angiotensinogen existing in plasma (Fig. 8).

As proposed above, angiotensinogen might be a substrate of NEP. Angiotensinogen could be cleaved directly to the product Ang(1-7) by NEP at the bond or position exactly the same as in AI between aminoacids proline and phenylalanine. From this proposal, the same renin substrate, angiotensinogen could also be cleaved by NEP. Thus, the amount of angiotensinogen remaining available for renin (for PRA assay) in plasma would be low (Fig. 8). The results from PRA obtained in this situation should be low (low renin). Therefore, question (3) can also be explained by this proposal.

Low renin: angiotensin-converting enzyme and Neutral endoptidase

In the renin-angiotensin system mechanism of hypertension, AII from ACE activity causing vasoconstriction is well documented. Another mechanism of hypertension, Ang(1-7) from the NEP activity causing water

* PRA: measure the amount of Ang I formation from its precursor substrate angiotensinogen by enzyme renin in plasma.

The enzyme activity depends on both the amounts of renin and substrate present and not just the amount of renin existed in plasma.

Thus, low PRA could also mean low amount of substrate angiotensinogen present in plasma and not necessarily only a low amount of enzyme renin in plasma.

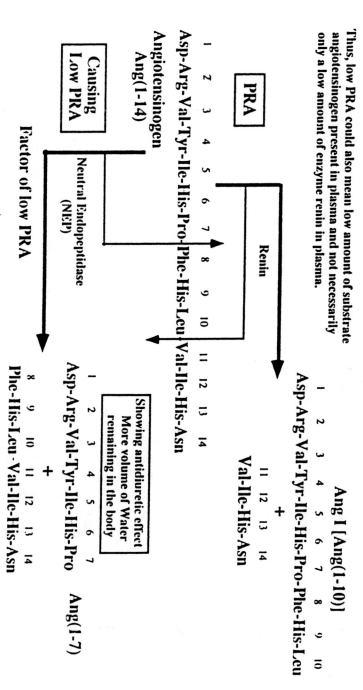

Fig. 8. The Cause of Low Plasma Renin Activity (PRA)*

retention, is a hypothetical concept. If patients have both mechanisms of hypertension, ACE inhibitor blocks the hypertension from vasoconstriction of the AII. A large amount of AI is built up in the presence of ACE inhibitor which is cleaved to Ang(1-7) by NEP. The hypertension from water retention occurs. In this case, the diuretic agent is required together with ACE inhibitor. Question (4) can also be nicely explained by this hypothetical proposal.

Using a diuretic agent is one approach for this kind treatment. It, however, is not the best way. Even using the diuretic agent to remove water, the mechanism of water retention still exists in the body. Therefore, abolishing the mechanism of water retention should be a better way. NEP inhibitor, such as SQ 28603 inhibits NEP activity to abolish the mechanism of water retention from the Ang(1-7) formed (Fig. 4). Simultaneously, it also blocks another water retention mechanism from the degradation of ANP by NEP (Fig. 5). However, no such drug is available yet for this kind of treatment. Treatment with either diuretic agent or NEP inhibitor alone without an ACE inhibitor present is also not good for these patients. Because the vasoconstriction mechanism from AII is still present, the blood pressure will still remain high.

Still, the mechanisms of water retention from the degradation of ANP and Ang(1-7) formation are different. They are from the same source of NEP activity (Fig. 4, 5 and 8). If NEP activity is inhibited, both mechanisms of water retention are simultaneously abolished.

As mentioned previously, some patients could not be treated with an ACE inhibitor because of itching and coughing from a large amount of bradykinin built up (Fig. 1 and 2). AII receptor antagonists should be used to substitute the ACE inhibitor. In low renin patients, AII receptor antagonist should also be used (instead of ACE inhibitor) together with diuretic agent for those patients who have an itching and coughing effect.

From the above explanation, hypertension can be summarized as follows. Hypertension results mainly from two important mechanisms, one from vasoconstriction and the other from water retention. Vasoconstriction is from AII by ACE activity. The water retention is from both the Ang(1-7) formation (hypothetical proposal) and ANP degradation both by NEP activity. AIII also contributes to the water retention. Both or either one of these mechanisms could occur in hypertensive patients. Treatment depends on which mechanism exists in the patients. ACE inhibitor or AII receptor antagonist can be used for the treatment of vasoconstricted hypertensive patients. Diuretic agent or NEP inhibitor can be used for the treatment of water retained hypertensive patients. Combination therapy should be used to treat both mechanisms operating in the patients. Treatment with diuretic agent to remove water does not necessarily mean the amount of water removed is enough to lower blood pressure. It also will remove the water from non-hypertensive persons or hypertensive persons without water retention mechanism. Using the NEP inhibitor from the start in combination therapy to abolish the mechanism of water retention should avoid this problem.

Combining the proposals from chapter I and II, the diagram of hypertension is assembled in Fig. 9. This diagram is a most completed picture for hypertension that is based on the relationship between the mechanisms of vasoconstriction and water retention. It is also related to the systolic pressure and diastolic pressure, respectively.

As shown in the diagram, inhibiting the ACE activity triggers the NEP to have higher activity and vice versa. Thus, the less response from vasoconstriction and more response from water retention and vice verse, respectively will be a result in hypertensive patients. Vasoconstriction and water retention for hypertention are related and influenced each other significantly in the renin-angiotensin system. Possibly, hypertension is a total result from the combination of vasoconstriction and water retention in renin-angiotensin system.

Conclusion

The causes of hypertension are mostly understood these days. Two major mechanisms for hypertension, vasoconstriction from AII and water retention, are well established. However, the relationship between each other and the mechanism of water retention are still not quite clear. One of the water retention mechanisms is also proposed from a hypothetical point of view. The relationship is connected well in most cases and the mechanism of water retention is made much clearer by the proposal from the concept.

The proposal is as follows:

(1) Water retention mechanism of hypertension besides AII vasocon-striction is also found from the same ACE substrate AI or renin substrate angiotensinogen.

(2) Water retention from the Ang(1-7) formation is a proposed hyperten-sive mechanism.

(3) Neutral endopeptidase (NEP) is the qualified enzyme proposed to cleave the substrates AI and angiotensinogen directly to Ang(1-7).

(4) Vasoconstriction and water retention are related and influence each other significantly.

(5) If the vasoconstriction response is higher in the system, then the water retention response must be lower and vice versa.

(6) Hypertension in renin-angiotensin system is a total result from the combination of vasoconstriction and water retention.

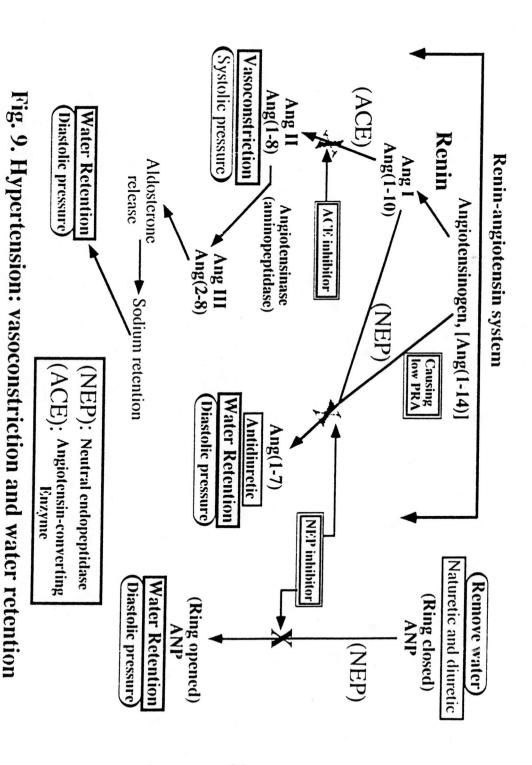

Fig. 9. Hypertension: vasoconstriction and water retention

Chapter III

Angiotensin-converting enzyme and its inhibitor

Angiotensin-converting enzyme (ACE) plays a very important role in hypertension. Angiotensin II (AII) is a potent vasoconstrictor in hypertensive disease. It is derived by the enzymatic cleavage action of ACE from its naturally occurring substrate angiotensin I (AI). The same enzyme also inactivates bradykinin (Fig. 1).

Blocking AII formation and bradykinin degradation by the enzymatic activity of ACE by using drugs such as captopril (Fig. 1) resulted in lowered blood pressure in many hypertensive patients. A historical account of the rational drug design via specific biochemical mechanism of this first ACE inhibitor, captopril, at the Squibb Institute is stated below.

A. Angiotensin-Converting Enzyme (ACE)

Skeggs and coworkers (1954) found that angiotensin was the pressor product of renin action known in hypertension. The product obtained from the incubation of renin with its plasma substrate in the presence of chloride was named angiotensin II. The product obtained in the absence of chloride was called angiotensin I. Angiotensin I was found to lack direct vasoconstriction action by studies in the artificially perfused kidney (Skeggs et al., 1956) and on the isolated aortic strip (Helmer, 1957). The enzyme responsible for the conversion of the inactive substrate angiotensin I to the active vasoconstrictor angiotensin II in the presence of chloride ion was partially purified from horse plasma by Skeggs et al. (1956), and was named angiotensin converting enzyme (originally hypertension converting enzyme). The enzyme appeared to contain a tightly bound functional metal ion, Zinc. From determination of the sequence of angiotensin I and II, apparently the angiotensin-converting enzyme hydrolyzed the carboxyl-terminal dipeptide His-Leu from the substrate decapeptide angiotensin I to liberate the biological active octapeptide angiotensin II (Lentz et al., 1956) (Fig. 1).

Substrate and Assays

Angiotensin I is a well known naturally occurring substrate for the angiotensin-converting enzyme (Skeggs et al., 1954; Skeggs et al..1956; Lentz et al., 1956). An understanding of the properties of angiotensin-converting enzyme was lacking. The chloride ion dependence, pH 7.5 optimum, metal ion and its products of dipeptide His-Leu and octapeptide angiotensin II from substrate angiotensin I were known properties. Angiotensin I was a specific substrate for angiotensin-converting enzyme. The structures of angiotensin I (decapeptide) and II (octapeptide) are Asp-Arg-Val-Tyr-Ile-His-Pro-Phe-His-Leu and Asp-Arg-Val-Tyr-Ile-His-Pro-Phe, respectively (Lentz, 1956; Cushman et al., 1981; Cheung, 1996) (Fig. 1).

Angiotensin I and II could be substrates for many other enzymes (Cheung, 1996), such as aminopeptidase, carboxypeptidase, neutral endopeptidase and others (Fig. 10). Using angiotensin I as substrate for measuring the true cleavage action from angiotensin-converting enzyme was impossible (Cheung, 1996). The amount of angiotensin II obtained was not a true and precise result. Thus, it might lead us to misunderstand angiotensin-converting enzyme.

To obtain the correct information and understand the properties of angiotensin-converting enzyme, purification of angiotensin-converting enzyme was one of the approaches. However, the purification procedure usually was very complicated and time consuming. The final yield was very small. The substrate AI was very expensive and large amounts need for use in vitro experiments was unavailable.

Shorter size substrate

Another approach was to modify the substrate angiotensin I from a longer size to a shorter size peptide that could be cleaved by angiotensin-converting enzyme the same way as substrate angiotensin I was cleaved. This shorter peptide must not be a substrate for some other enzymes. Even if you had the shorter peptide substrate of this kind, it required a new method for assaying the angiotensin-converting enzyme activity. Thus, the shorter peptide substrate allowed us to construct the model of angiotensin-converting enzyme and design inhibitors. It required only a very short period of time later for drug design.

Angiotensin I is a decapeptide with a dipeptide His-Leu and free carboxylic acid (-COOH) at its carboxyl-terminal (C-terminal) end of the peptide (Lentz, 1956; Cheung, 1996) (Figs. 1 and 10). Angiotensin-converting enzyme cleaves this C-terminal dipeptide His-Leu from the substrate angiotensin I and also liberates the another product angiotensin II (Figs. 1 and 10). The dipeptide is liberated from angiotensin-converting enzyme action instead of a single amino acid from carboxypeptidase action. Angiotensin-converting enzyme, thus, is an exopeptidase and classified as a carboxypeptidase (di-peptide carboxypeptidase, peptidyldipeptide carboxy hydrolase) (Cushman et al., 1981; Cheung, 1996).

Carboxypeptidase A and Hippuryl-Phenylalanine

Carboxypeptidase A (CPase A) is a different enzyme but similar to angiotensin-converting enzyme; it cleaves the substrate from its C-terminal end but only with the length of single amino acid (Fig. 11). The synthesized substrate of carboxypeptidase A was Hippuryl-Phenylalanine. Carboxypeptidase A cleaved the substrate Hippuryl-Phenylalanine (Fig. 11) to liberate the products of the single amino acid phenylalanine (C-terminal amino acid) and Hippuric acid (Hoffmann and Bergmann, 1940; Hartsuck and Lipscomb, 1971; Cheung, 1996).

Hippuryl-Histidyl-Leucine

The phenylalanine, single amino acid, in the structure of Hippuryl-Phenylalanine could be replaced by a dipeptide, Histidyl-Leucine, resulting in a compound, Hippuryl-Histidyl-Leucine (Hipp-His-Leu or HHL). HHL was proposed to be a specific synthetic shorter size substrate for ACE (Fig. 11) (Cushman and Cheung, 1971; Cheung, 1996). Hipp-His-Leu was also found to be cleaved by the angiotensin-converting enzyme in the same way that angiotensin I was cleaved (Fig. 11).

Angiotensin-converting enzyme would cleave both substrates, angiotensin I and Hipp-His-Leu, and produce two products for both substrates. The same dipeptide product His-Leu would be obtained from both substrates. Angiotensin II and Hippuric acid would then be the other products from the substrates, angiotensin I and Hipp-His-Leu, respectively (Fig.11).

41

Hipp-His-Leu was a synthetic substrate cleaved only by angiotensin-converting enzyme in the experimental conditions, because there were no other products found except the two expected products (Cushman and Cheung, 1971; Cheung, 1996).

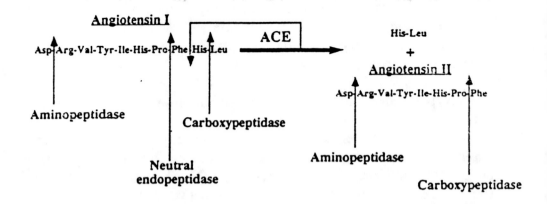

Fig. 10. Angiotensin I and II could be a substrate for many enzymes

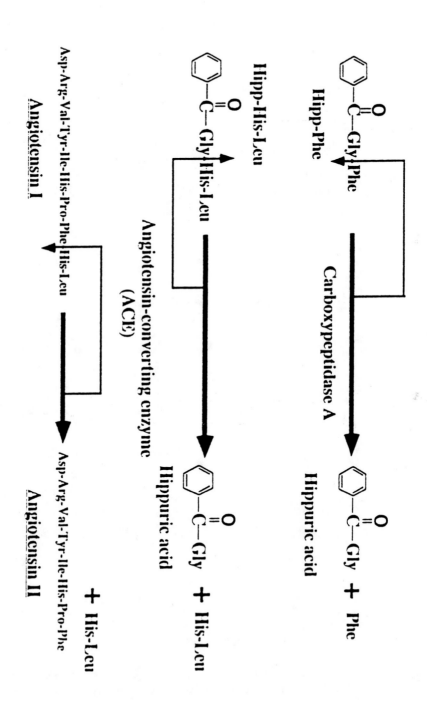

Fig. 11. The activities of carboxypeptidase A and angiotensin-converting enzyme

43

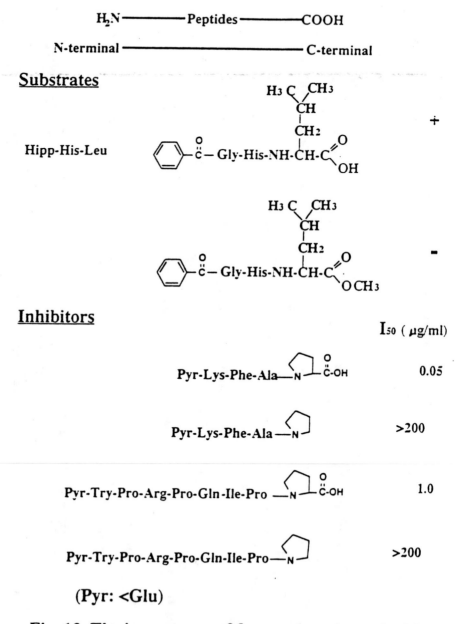

Fig. 12 The importance of free carboxyl terminal in
the structure of substrates and inhibitors

Properties of angiotensin-converting enzyme

The properties of angiotensin-converting enzyme obtained originally was based on the studies from the substrate angiotensin I (Ryan, et al., 1968; Boyd et al., 1969; Hollemans et al., 1969; Page et al., 1969; Dorer et al., 1970). As mentioned above, the chloride ion dependence, optimum pH 7.5, metal ion requirement and its activity liberating the products of dipeptide His-Leu and octapeptide angiotensin II from substrate angiotensin I were known properties. The optimal chloride concentration was found to be 0.03 M for the substrate Angiotensin I. The synthetic substrate Hipp-His-Leu was used to substitute for angiotensin I.

The properties of angiotensin-converting enzyme might have some changes and needed to be restudied with the substrate of Hipp-His-Leu. Indeed, the optimal chloride concentration and pH values were found shifted from 0.03 M and 7.5 to 0.3 M and 8.3, respectively (Cushman and Cheung, 1971). The liberated angiotensin II product was replaced by hippuric acid. The free carboxylic acid (-COOH) of the C-terminal in the structure is also required for the shorter size substrate (Fig. 12).

During pH optimum studies, the corrected pH curve and true pH optimum were difficult to obtain because the pH values shifted to a different number after chloride was added to the incubation solution. To overcome this problem, during buffer preparation, the pH was adjusted in the presence of 0.3 M NaCl (Cushman and Cheung, 1971). Thus, the pH curve and optimal pH values were obtained correctly (Cushman and Cheung, 1971).

Assay of Angiotensin-converting enzyme

The synthetic substrate Hipp-His-Leu was used as a substrate to replace angiotensin I for studying the cleavage action of angiotensin-converting enzyme (crude extract of rabbit lung acetone powder). Hippuric acid and His-Leu were the only two products from this angiotensin-converting enzyme action. In order to know how angiotensin-converting enzyme functioned, the amount of product of either Hipp or His-Leu must be measured.

The new assay developed for angiotensin-converting enzyme measured only the amount of Hippuric acid formed and not the His-Leu. We developed a method for measuring the product His-Leu fluorometrically but

45

not for this purpose. Hippuric acid could be directly determined spectro-photometrically at the wavelength of 228 nm (nanometer). However, Hipp-His-Leu could also be read at 228 nm together in the presence of Hippuric acid (Fig 13). Fortunately, Hippuric acid could be extracted into ethyl acetate organic solvent in the presence of HCl (hydrochloride) as a free acid form and thus, separated from Hipp-His-Leu as a salt form. The organic solvent ethyl acetate itself also could be read spectrophotometrically at 228 nm. The background reading from ethyl acetate was too high. The extracted Hippuric acid in ethyl acetate solution was evaporated to dryness in a heated Temp-Blok. The dried Hippuric acid was redissolved in water and the amount of Hippuric acid determined directly at 228 nm (Fig. 13).

Spectrophotometric assay of angiotensin-converting enzyme was as follows (Cushman and Cheung, 1971). The measure of Hipp-His-Leu hydrolysis by angiotensin-converting enzyme incubation was carried out at 37°C in disposable 13 X 100 mm tubes. Each 0.25 ml assay mixture contained the following components at the indicated final concentrations: potassium phosphate buffer (pH 8.3), 100 mm; sodium chloride, 300 mM; Hipp-His-Leu, 5 mM; and enzyme, 0-10 mU per 0.25 ml of assay volume. The enzyme, in a volume of 0.15 ml or less, was added last to initiate the enzyme reaction and tubes were incubated usually for 30 minutes, in a shaker water bath. One units of angiotensin-converting enzyme activity is defined at the amount catalyzing the formation of 1 μmole Hippuric acid from Hippuryl-His-Leu in 1 min. at 37°C under standard assay conditions.

The enzymic reactions are terminated by addition of 0.25 ml of 1 N HCl. The hippuric acid formed in the incubation is extracted into 1.5 ml ethyl acetate by vortex mixing. After a brief centrifugation, a 1.0 ml aliquot of each ethyl acetate layer is transferred to a clean tube. The extracted Hippuric acid in the ethyl acetate layer is evaporated by heating at 120°C for 30 min. in a Temp-Blok module heater. The dried hippuric acid is re-dissolved in 1.0 ml water and the amount of hippuric acid formed is deter-mined from its absorbance at 228 nm. (Fig. 13)

B. Drug Design

Synthesizing a compound (drug) is not that hard. Generating the idea of its correct structure is difficult. Searching for the idea is the function of drug design. It is also a way to know more about the enzyme.

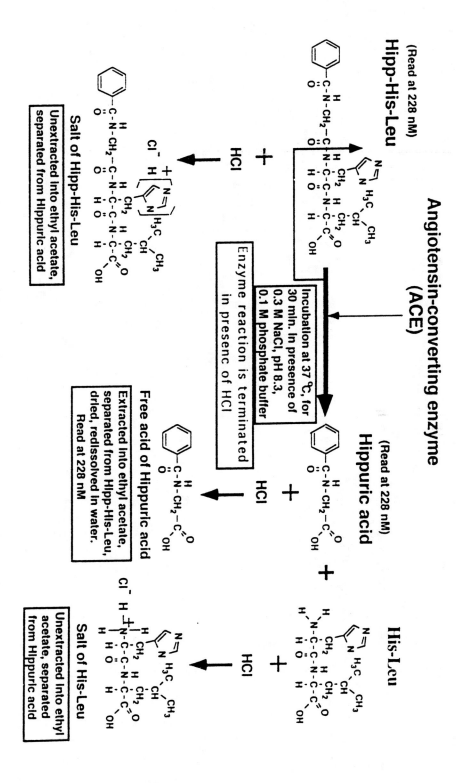

Fig. 13. Developed spectrophotometric assay of angiotensin-converting enzyme

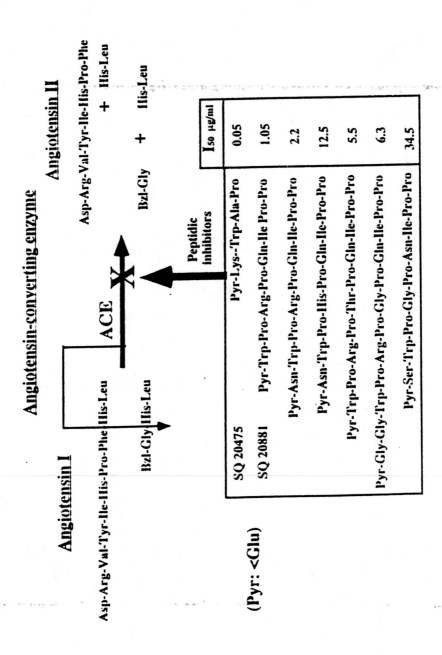

Fig. 14. Peptidic inhibitors from *Bothrops jararaca* venom

(Ferreira et al.,1970; Ondetti et al., 1971)

48

Requirements

The drug design of Angiotensin-converting enzyme inhibitors for hypertension required three important factors: (1) biochemical tool (2) methods and (3) knowledge. The biochemical tools and methods have been mentioned above, e.g., substrate Hipp-His-Leu and assay for angiotensin-converting enzyme, respectively (Cheung, 1996).

Relationship between substrate binding and enzyme activity

Specific knowledge regarding the active-site of angiotensin-converting enzyme would be crucial in drug design. The active-site of angiotensin-converting enzyme is the site at which substrate Ang I binds and is cleaved to produce products Ang II and His-Leu. Theoretically, substrate Ang I binding with ACE active-site first would precede the action of cleavage. If there were no binding, there would be no occurrence of this cleavage action of a substrate Ang I. Ang II formation from this action could not result. Hypertension from vasoconstriction also could not happen (Cheung, 1996).

Difference between substrate and inhibitor

The information of binding and cleavage (enzymatic catalytic action) is very important. Substrates differ from inhibitors, since substrates require both binding and enzymatic catalytic action (cleavage action for ACE) whereas inhibitors require only the binding. Substrate can function as an inhibitor for another different substrate of the same enzyme.

For inhibitor binding to ACE, a binding affinity between any inhibitor compound and ACE stronger than that of the substrate (Ang I or Hipp-His-Leu) would inhibit the formation of Ang II or Hippuric acid, respectively. In the end, Ang II or Hippuric acid were either completely stopped or produced in very small amounts (Cheung, 1996).

Relationship between inhibitor binding affinity and enzyme activity on the substrate

For measuring enzyme activity, it requires a measure of the amount of product formation (the ability of enzymatic catalytic action, such as cleavage action). The binding affinity of inhibitor with ACE, thus, could not be obtained from this study. The binding affinity between any enzyme, such as

ACE, and an inhibitor still can be accessed by the enzyme activity (cleavage activity for ACE) in the presence of inhibitor together with ACE and substrate. Theoretically, the stronger the inhibitor bound relative to the weaker binding ACE substrate, the more inhibitor would be bound and the less amount of substrate would be available for the cleavage action by enzyme. The enzyme activity would be very low. Thus, the binding affinity of inhibitor is indirectly proportional to the enzyme (ACE) activity (Cheung, 1996). Consequently, the stronger the binding affinity, the weaker the enzyme (ACE) activity is. Stronger binding affinity is referred to as inhibitor potency (I_{50}). The I_{50} is the concentration of inhibitor used to induce 50 % ACE blockade (50 % ACE activity). Higher I_{50} value of inhibitor indicates weaker inhibitor binding affinity with ACE (Cheung, 1996).

Snake venom inhibitors: SQ 20881 and SQ 20475

Snake venom inhibitors (Ferreira et al. 1970a and 1970b; Ondetti, et al., 1971; Stewart et al., 1971; Engel et al. 1972; Bakhle, 1972; Cushman and Cheung, 1972; Greene et al., 1972; Cheung and Cushman, 1973a and 1973b) (Fig. 14) were initially found as potent inhibitors for ACE. Two key inhibitor compounds from them, a nonapeptide (<Glu-Trp-Pro-Arg-Pro-Gln-Ile-Pro-Pro), SQ 20881 (teprotide) and a pentapeptide (<Glu-Lys-Trp-Ala-Pro), SQ 20475 (BPP$_{5a}$) were identified very early with the substrates Ang I and Hipp-His-Leu which led to the proposed ACE active site model (Cheung and Cushman, 1973a; Cheung and Cushman, 1973b; Cheung, 1996). The reason was that the information and results obtained from these 2 inhibitors for ACE were completely different and contrary. The detail is mentioned below. Thus, theirs bindings to ACE were confusing (Cheung, 1996). The free carboxylic acid in C-terminal was also required for the structure of inhibitors (Fig. 12).

Size of peptide inhibitor and substrate

I_{50} of SQ 20475 and SQ 20881 (Fig. 14 and 15) were 0.05 and 1.05 μg/ml (Cheung and Cushman, 1973a and 1973b; Cheung, 1996), respectively and suggested both bound well with ACE. However, the length of the structure of SQ 20881 was almost double the length of SQ 20475 (Fig 14 and 15). Why did these inhibitors bind well with ACE, even though, their sizes are completely different (Cheung and Cushman, 1973a and 1973b; Cheung 1996)? The binding of these 2 inhibitors to ACE had been studied further by testing the inhibition potency I_{50} of various analogs of these 2 compounds with either substitutions or shortening the size by one or more amino acids from the amino (N)-terminal end (Fig. 15) (Cheung and Cushman, 1973a and 1973b; Cushman et al., 1973; Cheung, 1996). The peptide that served as the substrate with a minimal size for the ACE presumed tripeptide length required the free carboxylic acid (-COOH) to be present at the carboxyl (C)-terminal end (Fig. 12 and 15).

Potent inhibitors SQ 20475 and SQ 20573 were not long-lasting

The presumed optimal tripeptide substrate sequences Trp-Ala-Pro and Phe-Ala-Pro appeared to be in the BPP_{5a} and SQ 20573 structures at the C-terminal end (Fig. 15). I_{50} of SQ 20573 was also found to be 0.05 µg/ml (Cheung and Cushman, 1973a and 1973b; Cushman et al. 1973) the same as SQ 20475. Both I_{50} values of SQ 20475 and SQ 20573 were better than the values of SQ 20881 and indicated that both SQ 20475 and SQ 20573 bound equally well and much more strongly than SQ 20881 with ACE. Even though, the binding of SQ 20475 and 20573 to ACE were stronger unfortunately such binding did not last long because they also served as substrates for ACE (Cheung, 1996). This was not the case, however, for SQ 20881. SQ 20881, even though, binding poorly could retain the inhibition potency for a long duration (Cheung, 1996).

Binding affinity from different sizes of peptide inhibitors

The I_{50} of both pentapeptides SQ 20475 and 20573 were identical and suggested both bound equally well with ACE. The only difference between these two pentapeptides: the tryptophan (Trp) in the center position of the structure of SQ 20475 was replaced by phenylalanine (Phe) to SQ 20573 (Fig 15). Thus, the C-terminal tripeptides of SQ 20475 and SQ 20573 Trp-Ala-Pro and Phe-Ala-Pro, respectively, also bound nearly well with ACE. It is a reasonable assumption. The C-terminal tripeptide of SQ 20881 was Ile-Pro-Pro. The I_{50} values of Ile-Pro-Pro (result based on <Glu-Ile-Pro-Pro), Trp-Ala-Pro (based on Phe-Ala-Pro) and Phe-Ala-Pro were found to be higher than 200, 1.4 and 1.4 µg/ml (Fig. 15), respectively. Thus, the C-terminal tripeptides of the shorter length of pentapeptides of SQ 20475 and SQ 20573 bound with ACE more favorably than the C-terminal tripeptide of longer length of nonapeptide of SQ 20881(Cheung and Cushman, 1973a and 1973b; Cheung, 1996). This information was also confusing: why SQ 20881 bound well with ACE, even though, its C-terminal tripeptide Ile-Pro-Pro

bound poorly (Cheung and Cushman, 1973a and 1973b; Cushman et al., 1973; Cheung, 1996).

Importance of Pro-Pro or Pro in the structure of C-terminal end

Even though, Pro-Pro also bound poorly (I_{50} value of 1,600 µg/ml) the presence of dipeptide Pro-Pro or single amino acid Pro at the C-terminal end could stop the enzymatic cleavage action at its C-terminal. The reason was the presence of a Pro having an imino bond attached at N atom of Pro substituted the amino bond at same position in the structure. Most enzymes cleave the amino bond (peptide bond) but not the imino bond (Fig. 16). The structure of the compound with an imino bond present at the cleavage position, thus, could abolish enzyme cleavage action. Therefore, the C-terminal dipeptide Pro-Pro or single amino acid Pro was deemed very important especially for an inhibitor which bound ACE poorly. The shorter size structure (SQ 20475 or SQ 20573) bound tighter with ACE than the longer size of SQ 20881. Even though, they were inhibitors, they could also be substrate for ACE because an amino bond was present at the cleavage position of the structure by ACE. The longer size of structure SQ 20881 has an imino bond (-Pro-Pro) at the cleavage position of the C-terminal end. It bound worse than short size structures, but could only be an inhibitor for ACE. The imino bond present in the structure of SQ 20881 at the cleavage position will stop the enzymatic cleavage action and stabilizes this compound (Cheung, 1996) (Fig. 15). As a result of this stabilization for the compound existing in the environmental conditions, this compound therefore served as an inhibitor.

Fixed size of ACE active-site, varied sizes of peptide inhibitors

Generally speaking, every thing has its own fixed length size including chemical compounds, substrates, inhibitors, enzymes and ACE active-site. Substrates and inhibitors are bound to the ACE active-site (Cheung, 1996). Thus, the various sizes of substrates or inhibitors in relevance to the fixed size of the active-site play an important role in the binding as well. The size of SQ 20881 was much greater than the size of SQ 20475, but, both possibly fit into the same pocket of the ACE active-site. From the results above, the I_{50} value of Trp-Ala-Pro was just as good as SQ 20881. It strongly indicated that the substrate which had the size of a tripeptide that bound to ACE, were just as tight as the size of nonapeptide SQ 20881 (Cheung, 1996) (Fig. 15).

Issues

Those issues remained to confound the observations as mentioned above: (1) How could SQ 20881 bind very well to ACE even though its C-terminal tripeptide Ile-Pro-Pro did bind poorly? (2) That the relevant size of SQ 20881 appeared to be possibly disproportional than the ACE active-site. (3) A short tripeptide Trp-Ala-Pro would bind as efficiently as a very long peptide SQ 20881. Those issues might suggest that SQ 20881 bound well with ACE but might not be bound at the same site as SQ 20475. However, from enzyme kinetic studies, all inhibitors and substrates including Ang I, Hipp-His-Leu, SQ 20881 and SQ 20475 bound with ACE exactly at the same site. Thus, the model of the ACE active-site was confusing and hard to picture (Cheung, 1996).

Proposal

In the early 70's, I proposed a simplistic model of the ACE active-site after 2 years of effort in pursuit of above issues (Cheung and Cushman, 1973b;). In September 1996, a specific binding concept from the mechanical view to propose the model of the ACE active site that has aided the ACE inhibitor drug development was published (Cheung, 1996) in the "BIO/PHARMA Quarterly." This mechanical view is also presented here in this article.

(a) A mechanical view of the specific ACE binding Model (Fig. 17):

An analogy was used to present the specific model idea. Two pieces of wood, one long and the other short, are tied together with electrical tape. They are tied together very well at the positions of the two ends of the short wood (see Fig. 17, top two pictures). In this case, the middle portion of the long wood is heavily coated with oil. This long wood cannot be tied together with short wood at this oily position. The other end still binds to the long wood well. The binding of the short piece to the long piece of wood, thus, is poor (Fig. 17, middle 3 pictures). For tightening purposes, attaching another piece of wood to the short wood will extent the wood length beyond the oily position of the long wood. The free end of the wood extension can thus bind to the long wood but at a different position without oil presence. This extension can make the entire piece bind tightly to the long wood (Fig. 17, bottom two pictures) (Cheung, 1996).

(b) Constructed ACE active-site binding model (Fig. 18)

Using this mechanical view allowed constructing of the ACE active-site binding model (Cheung, 1996). The long wood represents ACE active-site. The short wood (or with extension) represents the peptide inhibitors or substrates. The binding of this long and short wood (or with extension) is just like the binding of the ACE active-site and substrate or inhibitor together, respectively. The extension piece whether required or not depends on how well the short wood is bound to the long wood. For inhibitor binding to the ACE active-site, the requirement of extension size of the inhibitor (longer size peptide inhibitor) also depends on how well the shorter size C-terminal di or tripeptide bound to the ACE active-site (Cheung, 1996).

The specific model of the active-site of ACE contains 2 portions connecting to each other.

(1) The essential binding and cleavage site (EBCS): the C-terminal tripeptide of substrate or inhibitor must bind at this site. The free (-COOH) of a molecule has to initiate binding at this site and then aligns each remaining group of the molecule to either bind or fit in the right pocket of the ACE active-site. A Zinc (Zn) ion is at this site and is involved with the length of dipeptide in the substrate binding and cleavage. The EBCS is the predominate site for ACE cleavage activity (Cheung and Cushman, 1973b; Cheung, 1996).

(2) The Auxiliary binding site (ABS): when the binding of the C-terminal tripeptide of a substrate or inhibitor at EBCS is poor, the remaining molecule beyond the tripeptide region is required and is going to bind at this ABS to enhance the binding of the whole molecule of the inhibitor or the substrate with ACE (Cheung and Cushman, 1973b; Cheung, 1996).

		I_{50} (μg/ml)
	H₂N ——————— Peptides ——————— COOH	
	N-terminal ——————————————— C-terminal	
SQ 20475	Pyr-Lys-Trp-Ala-Pro	0.05
SQ 20573	Pyr-Lys-Phe-Ala-Pro	0.05
	Lys-Phe-Ala-Pro	1.2
	Phe-Ala-Pro	1.4
	Ala-Pro	50.00
	Pyr-Lys-Phe-Ala-Ala	0.06
	Pyr-Lys-Phe-Pro-Pro	3.3
	Pyr-Lys-Ile-Ala-Pro	1.6
	Pyr-Nle-Phe-Ala-Pro	0.2
	Pyr-Trp-Pro-Arg-Pro	14.0
SQ 20881	Pyr-Trp-Pro-Arg-Pro-Gln-Ile-Pro-Pro	1.1
	Pro-Arg-Pro-Gln-Ile-Pro-Pro	10
	Arg-Pro-Gln-Ile-Pro-Pro	32
	Z-Pro-Gln-Ile-Pro-Pro	80
	Pyr-Ile-Pro-Pro	> 200
	Pyr-Phe-Pro-Arg-Pro-Gln-Ile-Pro-Pro	2.8
	Pyr-Trp-Pro-Lys-Pro-Gln-Ile-Pro-Pro	1.5
	Pyr-Trp-Pro-Arg-Pro-Gln-Phe-Pro-Pro	0.3
	Pyr-Trp-Pro-Arg-Pro-Gln-Ile-Ala-Pro	0.4

(Pyr: <Glu)

Fig. 15. Structure relationship of synthetic peptidic inhibitors

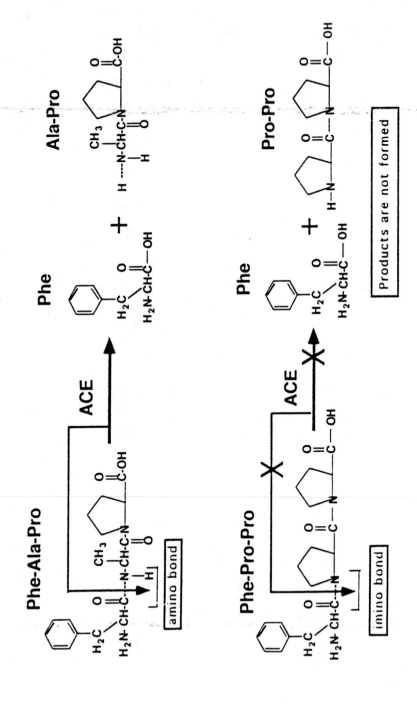

Fig. 16. Difference of amino and imino bond for enzymes

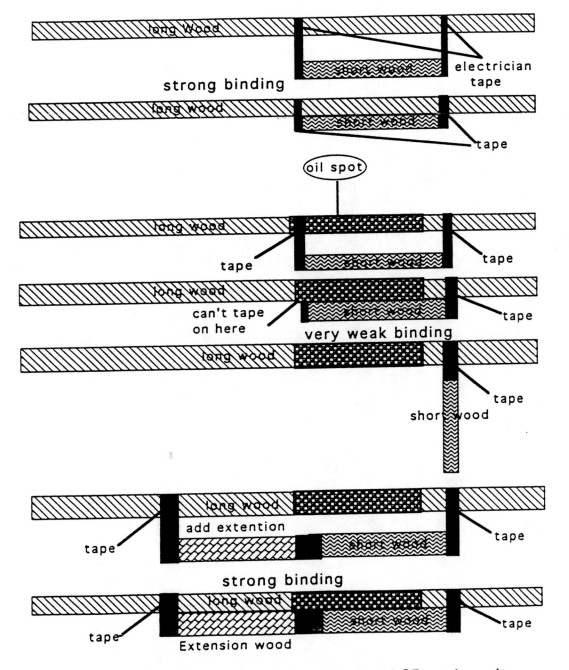

Fig. 17. Mechanical view for proposing ACE active-site

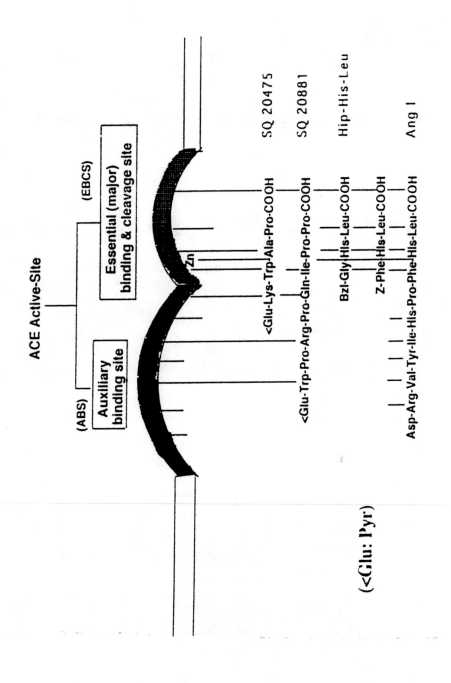

Fig. 18.

Hypothetical model of active-site of Angiotensin-converting enzyme

58

The above specific binding model of ACE action can explain why SQ 20881 and SQ 20475 having different length size do not bind the same way with ACE, but, both bind well with ACE at the same site. It also explains all other remaining issues and questions well.

(c) Angiotensin-converting enzyme inhibitor design

ACE Inhibitor Drug Development

During the early search for a lead compound for therapeutic use, SQ 20881 was identified from the components of the venom of a Brazilian viper, *Bothrops jararaca* (Cheung and Cushman, 1973a and 1973b; Cushman et al., 1973; Cheung, 1996) as a first potent and long lasting active inhibitor (drug) for ACE and hypertensive disease. However, it was found to be not orally active and very expensive to make. Various size peptides and orally active inhibitors have been synthesized since. From the active-site model, the inhibitor size and configuration as a single amino acid, dipeptide, tripeptide or even longer were examined (Cheung, 1996). The configurations of dipeptide analogs were considered as product inhibitors (product: dipeptide). Configuration with tripeptide analogs or longer were considered as substrate inhibitor (substrate: tripeptide or longer) (Cheung, 1996).

Dipeptide inhibitors, dicarboxylic acids (SQ 13745) and (SQ 13297)

Due to C-terminal tripeptide Phe-Ala-Pro of SQ 20573, this inhibitor bound to ACE just as well as the longer size nonapeptide SQ 20881. The dipeptide was the product of the substrate from ACE action. Shorter peptide inhibitor would be considered highly for synthesis. We concentrated only on the product (dipeptide) inhibitors. It was initially from and focused on the compound benzylsuccinic acid (dicarboxylic acid) (Byers and Wolfenden, 1972 and 1973) (Fig. 19), a carboxypeptidase A (CPase A) synthetic inhibitor, and thus, the compound succinyl-L-proline (SQ 13745) (Fig. 19) was synthesized (Cushman et al., 1977,1978 and 1979; Ondetti, et al. 1977) for ACE as a dipeptide (product) inhibitor.

Benzylsuccinic acid is an analog of single amino acid phenylalanine, that is the product from the substrate Hippuryl-Phenylalanine (Hipp-Phe) by CPase A (Fig. 11). It was considered as a product inhibitor of CPase A As mentioned above, CPase A is an enzyme similar to ACE. It cleaves the C-terminal single amino acid only instead of dipeptide from ACE action. The

Succinyl-L-Pro (dicarboxylic acid) is also an analog of dipeptide Gly-Pro (Fig. 19). It was also considered as a product inhibitor for ACE because it has the configuration of Gly-Pro (dipeptide) (Cheung, 1996). The I_{50} of SQ 13745 for ACE was 135 µg/ml (Fig. 20) (Cushman et al., 1977,1978 and 1979; Ondetti, et al. 1977; Cheung, 1996). It would bind to ACE poorly.

Ala-Pro is the product from the most important potent inhibitors (SQ 20475 or 20573) or substrate (its C-terminal Trp-Ala-Pro or Phe-Ala-Pro) which has a very strong binding affinity with ACE at EBCS. The analog of Ala-Pro is α-D-methyl-succinyl-L-proline. Succinyl-Proline was replaced to α-D-methyl-succinyl-L-proline (or D-2-methyl-succinyl-L-proline, SQ 13297) with I_{50} at 12 µg/ml (Fig. 20) (Cushman et al., 1977,1978 and 1979; Ondetti, et al. 1977; Cheung, 1996). The binding was 11 times better but still not satisfactory. After extensive studies of the analogs of SQ 13297 and 13745 with one or more carbon length increased or removed or addition of extra groups in the succinyl moiety (Fig. 21), it was found that it didn't help the binding significantly. Thus, the binding of the free carboxyl group (-COOH) in the succinyl portion to the ACE at EBCS with Zinc must be not too strong (Cheung, 1996).

Importance of the binding between Zinc and Sulfur

The substitution of the carboxyl group on an inhibitor might be significant for improving Zn binding. Numerous chemical groups had been studied to replace the carboxylic acid group. It was found that the sulfhydryl group (-SH) bound to the Zn very tightly (Cushman et al., 1977, 1978 and 1979; Ondetti, et al. 1977; Cheung, 1996). To make a point for easy understanding (Cheung, 1996), as one would see in a qualitative analytical chemistry experiment in an university's laboratory, bubbling hydrogen sulfide gas (H_2S) into a divalent metal ion solution would result in a black precipitate in the solution (Fig. 22). Zn is the divalent metal ion in the solution. The black precipitate in this solution is zinc sulfide (ZnS) (Fig. 22). Thus, Zn and sulfur bind extremely well. Its solubility product of 1.2×10^{-23} (Fig. 22) also indicates the strong binding.

Dipeptide inhibitor, sulfhyldryl analogs (SH) of dipeptides (SQ 14225 and SQ 13863)

The -SH substitution for the carboxyl group (-COOH) in the succinyl portion of the SQ 13297 and SQ 13745 would be a very significant advance in the development of an ACE inhibitor. The S-substituted compound of SQ 13745 was SQ13863 (3-mercaptopropanoyl-L-Proline) and resulted in an I_{50} value of 0.05 μg/ml against ACE (Fig. 23) (Cushman et al., 1977,1978 and 1979; Ondetti, et al. 1977; Cheung, 1996). As a result of this -SH substitution for the -COOH in the same position of the same compound SQ 13745, it made the binding with Zn at EBCS site 2700 times stronger. Logically, the S-substituted compound of the more favorable binding configuration of dipeptide Ala-Pro, SQ 14225 (D-3-mercapto-2-methyl propanoyl-L-Proline) would result in another about 10 times better binding than SQ 13863 based on the I_{50} values from both SQ 13297 and SQ 13745. Indeed, the I_{50} value of SQ 14225 was 0.005 μg/ml (Fig. 23) (Cushman et al., 1977, 1978 and 1979; Ondetti, et al., 1977; Cheung, 1996). That the binding of SQ 14225 was found to be 10 times better than SQ 13863 resulted from the additional methyl group in the propanoyl at the 2 position. The binding of SQ 14225 thus, was 27,000 times (by weight) or 35,000 times (by mole) stronger (potent) than SQ 13745 (Cheung, 1996).

CAPOTEN®, captopril

These two new compounds were further elucidated in the series of ACE inhibitor searches. SQ 14225 was found to be 200 times more potent (by weight) and 60 times (by mole) than SQ 20881, teprotide, based on the I_{50} value. The binding affinity of SQ 14225 with ACE was also considered about 60 times stronger than SQ 20881. The binding of SQ 14225 with the active-site of the angiotensin-converting enzyme is shown in Fig. 24. SQ 14225 was also found to be orally active and developed for human hypertensive disease. SQ 13863 was not pursued further. SQ 14225

$$\overset{\displaystyle CH_3}{\underset{\displaystyle |}{}}$$

has a chemical structure of **HS-CH₂-CH-CO-Proline** (Fig. 25) (Cushman et al., 1977,1978 and 1979; Ondetti, et al. 1977; Cheung, 1996). and has been named captopril, or CAPOTEN®.

Amino acid

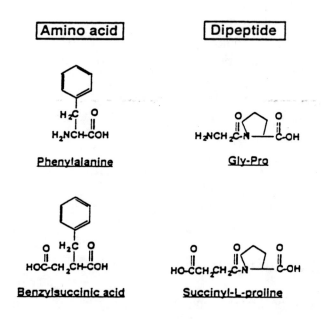

H₂C O
H₂NCH-COH

Phenylalanine

Dipeptide

H₂NCH₂C-N──C-OH

Gly-Pro

O H₂C O
HOC-CH₂CH-COH

Benzylsuccinic acid

HO-CCH₂CH₂-N──C-OH

Succinyl-L-proline

Fig. 19. Configuration of an amino acid, a dipeptide and their analogs

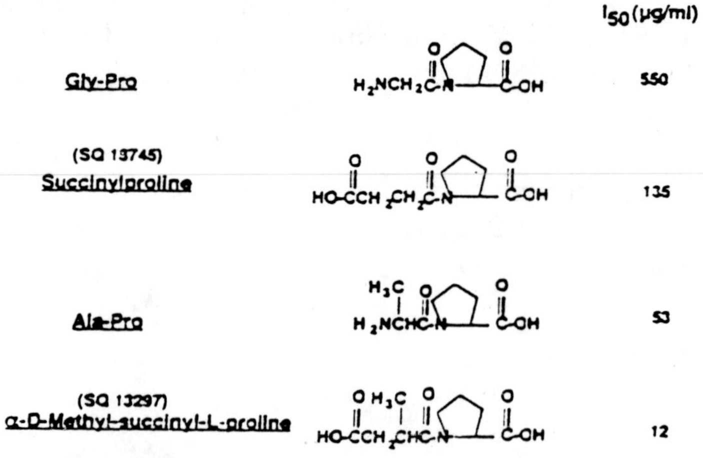

I_{50} (µg/ml)

Gly-Pro

H₂NCH₂C-N──C-OH

550

(SQ 13745)
Succinylproline

HO-CCH₂CH₂-N──C-OH

135

Ala-Pro

H₂NCHC-N──C-OH

53

(SQ 13297)
α-D-Methyl-succinyl-L-proline

HO-CCH₂CHC-N──C-OH

12

Fig. 20. ACE inhibition by dipeptides and their analogs

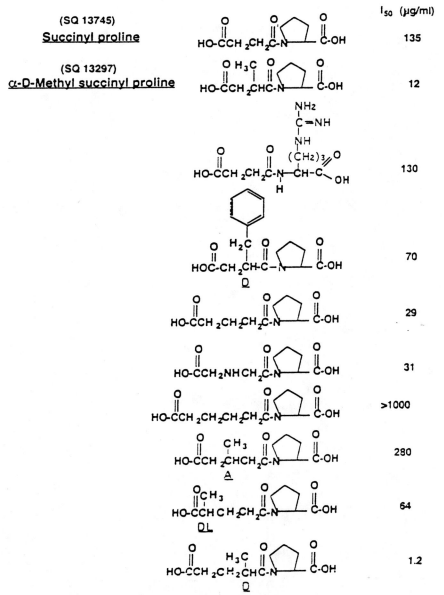

Fig. 21. ACE inhibition by the inhibitors of various dicarboxylic acids

Qualitative analytical chemistry

$$M^{++} \; + \; S^- \longrightarrow MS \downarrow$$

$$ZnCl_2 \; + \; H_2S \longrightarrow ZnS \downarrow \; + \; 2\,HCl$$

Solubility product of ZnS: $\quad 1.25 \times 10^{-23}$

Fig. 22. Chemical equation of di-valence metal ion with sulfide

		I_{50} (μg/ml)
SQ 13745 Succinyl proline	HO-C CH$_2$CH$_2$C-N—C-OH	135
SQ 13863 3-mercaptopropanoyl -L-proline	HSCH$_2$CH$_2$C-N—C-OH	0.05
SQ 13297 α-D-methylsuccinyl-L-proline	HO-C CH$_2$CHC-N—C-OH	12
SQ 14225 D-3-mercapto-2-methyl propanoyl-L-proline	HSCH$_2$CHC-N—C-OH	0.005

Fig. 23. ACE inhibition by the sulfhdryl and carboxyl inhibitors

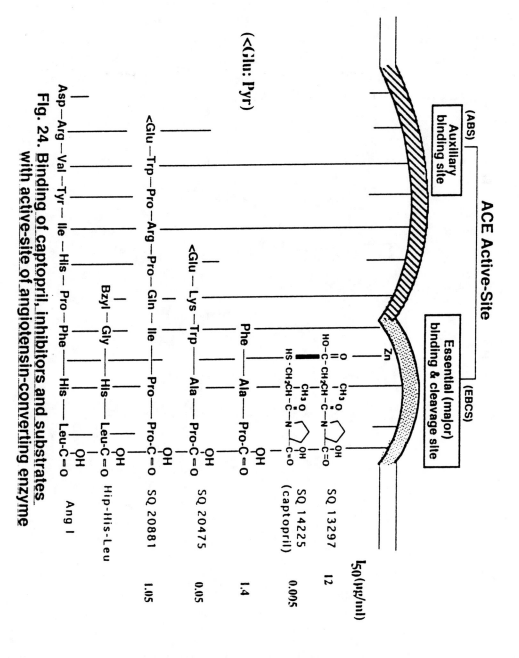

Fig. 24. Binding of captopril, inhibitors and substrates with active-site of angiotensin-converting enzyme

65

Conclusion

Captopril is a potent ACE inhibitor, the *first* orally active antihypertensive ACE inhibitor drug. Its design began with a hypothesis that AII might be involved in the pathogenesis of hypertension. In a process of constructing the hypothesis to the full development of an antihypertensive drug, from a stage of invisible unknowns to a clearly visible picture, it had allowed us to achieve the goal of generating a drug by rational design. *Captopril was the true breakthrough drug in drug development history.*

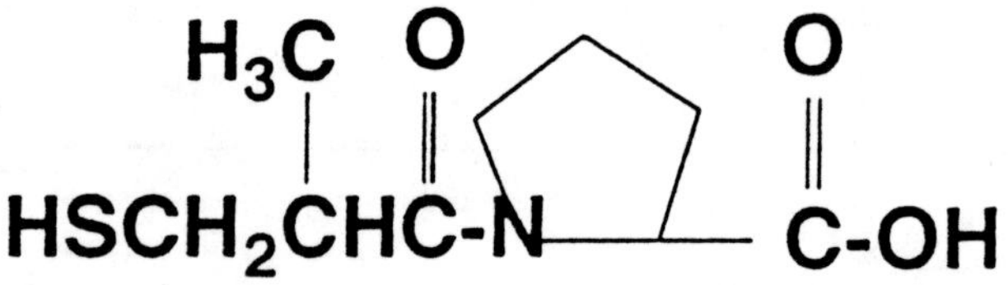

$$H_3C \quad O \qquad\qquad O$$

$$HSCH_2CHC-N \underset{}{\bigtriangleup} C-OH$$

Captopril   (capoten®)

SQ 14225

Fig 25. Structure of captopril

Chapter IV

Thoughts for drug making

Enzyme's point of view

The design of captopril came from the binding concept between enzyme and inhibitor. The requirement as inhibitor for enzyme will depend on the enzyme's view (Cheung, 1996). Many synthetic compounds for ACE inhibition studies including captopril (SQ 14225) and other synthetic ACE inhibitor drugs on the market are nonpeptide compounds. From the enzyme's point view, they all are bound the same way as the configuration of peptides with ACE, and are considered and classified as peptide inhibitors.

Tripeptide inhibitor

Captopril has a dipeptide configuration as ACE inhibitor hypertensive drug. As mentioned in the above chapter, from the ACE active-site model, the compound size and configuration as single amino acid, dipeptide, tripeptide or even longer size could be inhibitor (Cheung, 1996). The tripeptide compound was also known as inhibitor in the early research period such as Phe-Ala-Pro with I_{50} value of 1.4 µg/ml. As discussed earlier, minimal size of a peptide to be a substrate is tripeptide. The tripeptide inhibitor Phe-Ala-Pro was found also as a substrate for ACE. The I_{50} value of 1.4 µg/ml, therefore, was not corrected for Phe-Ala-Pro. The reason was that Phe-Ala-Pro during the inhibition study in the incubation some amount was cleaved to two products of Phe and Ala-Pro by ACE. The available amount of inhibitor was not the same amount that we supposed. Obviously, the binding affinity of Phe-Ala-Pro should be much better. Thus, Phe-Ala-Pro structure can be modified in the bond between Phe and Ala to another new compound which cannot be cleaved by ACE. Theoretically, the binding affinity of this new proposed compound, if it still retained the original tripeptide configuration of Phe-Ala-Pro would be very strong with ACE. The bond ACE cleaved between Phe and Ala in Phe-Ala-Pro is a peptide bond (-CO-NH-). As a result of the modification from theory, this peptide bond (-CO-NH-) changes to the non-peptide bond, either (-CH$_2$-NH-) or (-CO-CH$_2$-) and will stabilize the bond without cleavage by ACE. The tripeptide configurations of this new modified compound (Cheung, 1996, 1997) are shown in Fig. 26.

Another approach to have the configuration of tripeptide of a new modified compound was strictly based from building the structures of molecular models of three different compounds. Phe-Ala-Pro with the best binding affinity to ACE (I_{50} value of 1.4 μg/ml) was in the configuration of tripeptide compounds. The SQ 13297 α-D-methyl succinyl proline was found to be a compound of dipeptide configuration in the dicarboxylic acid structure having stronger binding affinity with ACE.

One compound, glutarylproline, (Fig. 21) with one carbon length increased in the structure of SQ 13745, was an I_{50} value of 29 μg/ml; its binding affinity was a little worse than SQ 13297 but about 4.7 times stronger than SQ 13745. Its size is little longer and shorter than the configuration of dipeptide and tripeptide, respectively.

By building the molecular structure models from Dreiding stereo-models, three different structure models were obtained for the above three compounds. These three structure models were aligned with each other for each corresponding group, initiated from the free carboxylic group of the C-terminal and then tied together with string to become a new modified structure model in the configuration of a tripeptide (Fig. 27)

The configuration of the tripeptide structure above was proposed in the early 70's (Fig. 26 and 27), and had the structures of a tripeptide inhibitor (remarkably similar to the compound, enalaprilat) (Cheung, 1996, 1997). However, a compound as such was not synthesized.

Dipeptide used as a tool

Searching for the best configuration of inhibitor for binding with enzyme is very hard and time consuming. It is impossible for the chemist to make every compound available for this kind of study. In the middle 70's, we tried to optimize configuration of peptide inhibitors. Alternatively, using available compounds already on the market could prove the point for this study. ACE cleaves the dipeptide from its C-terminal substrate. The configuration of dipeptide inhibitor (it is not necessarily a dipeptide compound) has already been studied. The best configuration of the dipeptide as inhibitor was still unclear. That information could be obtained from studies using all dipeptide compounds available on the market. Dipeptides were separated into three major categories (Cheung et al. 1980) (Fig. 28). In the first two categories, the amino acid glycine was fixed either in N-terminal or C-terminal of the dipeptide structure. The remaining amino acid was varied in the other position of the dipeptide structure (Glycyl-AA or AA-Glycine, respectively, AA: amino acid). The third category, both amino acids either in C-terminal or N-terminal position of the dipeptide were varied (AA-AA) (Cheung et al., 1980).

As a result of these studies (Cheung et al., 1980), the favorable configuration of the amino acid in either C-terminal or N-terminal in the structure of the dipeptide would be obtained (Fig. 28). The range of the I_{50} values for the Gly-AA (Fig. 28) was from 30 to 9600 μM (300-fold difference). Gly-Trp was found the best configuration with I_{50} of 30 μM in this series. Gly-Pro was found to be 15 times worse than the Tryptophan (Trp) in the proline position in the dipeptide with I_{50} of 450 μM. In the AA-Gly (Fig. 28), the range of the I_{50} values found was from 1,100 to 17,000 μM (15.5-fold difference). The best and worst were the Val-Gly and Pro-Gly, respectively. The binding of Ala-Gly was close to the best Val-Gly with I_{50} of 2,500 μM. Combining both best binding amino acids from N- and C-terminal to a dipeptide was Val-Trp. The binding of Val-Trp, theoretically, from these studies would be the best configuration in the dipeptide structure. Ala-Pro was the configuration of dipeptide from the known ACE inhibitor SQ 14225 (captopril). As a result obtained from the dipeptide of both amino acids varied in their corresponding position, the Val-Trp indeed was found to be the best in binding (I_{50} of 1.6 μM) (Fig. 28). Ile-Phe turned out to be the worst (I_{50} of 930 μM) for binding of a dipeptide structure. Surprisingly, the binding of Ala-Pro was poor (I_{50} of 230 μM). The proline in the end of C-terminal peptide inhibitor or substrate was already known to bind poorly to ACE from the information of ACE properties. The binding of Pro-Pro would be even worse with I_{50} of 6400 μM (1600 μg/ml) (Fig. 28).

To predict the better binding configuration in drug design, the I_{50} values of Gly-AA (NH_2-CH_2-CO-AA) dipeptides have been compared with the I_{50} values of its SH derivative of Gly-AA (HS-CH_2-CH_2-CO-AA) (Cheung et al. 1980) (Fig. 29). The class of SH compounds (mercapto-propanoyl amino acids) are much better binding (more potent) inhibitors of angiotensin-converting enzyme than are the class of the Gly-AA dipeptides. Similar relative bindings with angiotensin-converting enzyme are found with the

69

identical amino acid residues in the structure of the C-terminal among the members of the two classes of inhibitors. The preliminary studies indicated that the portions of the amino acids in the Gly-AA dipeptide compound that are favorable towards binding with ACE are also found to similarly enhance the binding relationship for the identical amino acid portions in the class of SH compounds (Fig. 29). Trp is the best in both classes of the inhibitors. Pro and Phe are second and third, respectively, also in both classes. Aspartic acid is the worst in both classes. As a result of this study, it suggested that using a dipeptide as a tool might be of great aid in the design of favorable binding portions of enzyme inhibitors. This method has been used by Dr. Liorens, et al. (1980) and Dr. Roques, et al. (1980). Thiorphan, therefore, was found to be the best binding configuration of the dipeptide inhibitor for enkephalinease in their studies at that time.

Different concept in drug development

Drug design can be from many different methods. Rational design is one of the routes proven to have a breakthrough drug, such as captopril. Screening old and new synthesized compounds may find a new application or different treatment for that compound. Screening natural products and herbs may find different drugs and different applications in treatment. The new technology of molecular biology may be a great help for new drug design.

Two drugs (or more) mixed together

Two (more) different drugs also can be mixed together for either the same treatment or two (more) different treatments simultaneously. The mixture of drugs has been used already in patients, such as those with low renin hypertension. Two different drugs are two different compounds, one only for each corresponding treatment. To use less different kinds of drugs in patients, one single compound (drug) used simultaneously for different treatments can be of more benefit to patients.

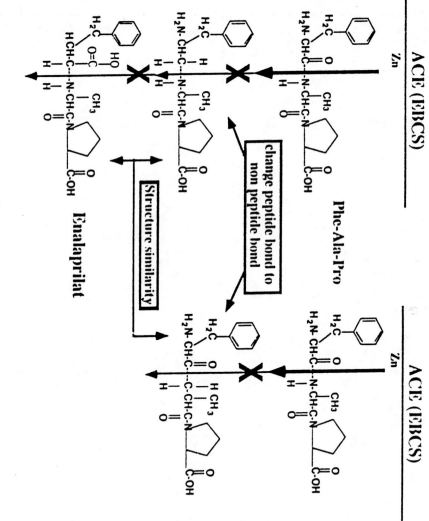

Fig. 26. Tripeptide configuration model of ACE inhibitor (A)

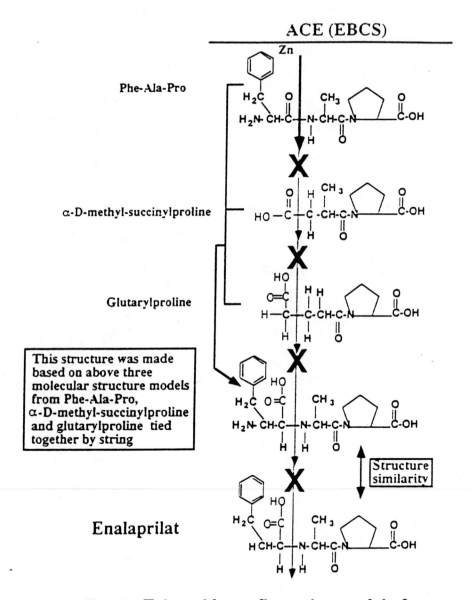

Fig. 27. Tripeptide configuration model of
ACE inhibitor (B)

Dipeptide Gly-AA*	I_{50}(μM)	Dipeptide *AA-Gly	I_{50}(μM)	Dipeptide *AA-AA*	I_{50}(μM)
Gly-Trp	30	Val-Gly	1,100	Val-Trp	1.6
Gly-Tyr	210	Ile-Gly	1,200	Ile-Trp	2.0
Gly-Pro	450	Arg-Gly	1,200	Ile-Tyr	3.7
Gly-Phe	630	Tyr-Gly	2,000	Ala-Trp	10
Gly-Ile	1,200	Ala-Gly	2,500	Arg-Trp	16
Gly-Met	1,400	Lys-Gly	3,200	Val-Tyr	22
Gly-Ala	2,000	Phe-Gly	3,700	Val-Phe	53
Gly-Leu	2,500	Met-Gly	4,300	Ala-Tyr	88
Gly-His	3,100	Trp-Gly	5,900	Ile-Pro	130
Gly-Arg	3,200	His-Gly	6,300	Arg-Pro	130
Gly-Ser	3,800	Gly-Gly	7,200	Ala-Phe	190
Gly-Val	4,600	Gln-Gly	7,400	Ala-Pro	230
Gly-Lys	5,400	Ser-Gly	8,500	Arg-Phe	230
Gly-Glu	5,400	Leu-Gly	8,800	Val-Pro	420
Gly-Thr	5,700	Thr-Gly	9,900	Ile-Phe	930
Gly-Gln	7,000	Glu-Gly	10,000	Pro-Pro	6400
Gly-Gly	7,200	Asp-Gly	14,000		
Gly-Asp	9,600	Pro-Gly	17,000		

* AA: Amino acid

Fig. 28. Inhibition of angiotensin-converting enzyme by dipeptides

AA*: Amino Acid	$I_{50}(\mu M)$ Gly-AA* dipeptide (NH$_2$-CH$_2$-CO-AA)	$I_{50}(\mu M)$ Mercaptopropanoyl-AA* (SH-CH$_2$-CH2-CO-AA)
Tryptophan	30	0.07
Proline	450	0.20
Phenylalanine	630	0.40
Alanine	2000	0.85
Leucine	2500	1.60
Arginine	3200	1.70
Lysine	5400	2.40
Glycine	7200	3.20
Aspartic acid	9200	68.00

Fig. 29. The relationship between dipeptide Gly-AA and thiol analogs of dipeptide (SH-CH2-CH2-CO-AA) from the inhibition of angiotensin-converting enzyme

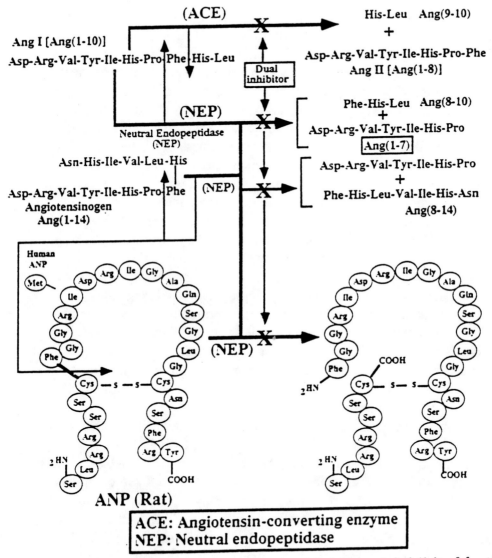

Fig. 30. One single compound (dual inhibitor) inhibited both
enzymes: angiotensin-converting enzyme and
neutral endopeptidase

Two different enzyme inhibitors synthesized in one single compound

An ACE inhibitor (captopril) is a drug for hypertensive patients. In low renin hypertensive patients, the effect of captopril for lowering the blood pressure was not good. Using capozide instead of captopril was very effective. CAPOZIDE® (registered trademark of Bristol-Myers Squibb, Inc.) is a mixture of two compounds, captopril and hydrocholorothiazide (HCTZ). Captopril is an ACE inhibitor. HCTZ is a diuretic. Diuretic drugs are known for removing water from the body. However, the water retention mechanism is still present in the body even when using diuretics. To stop the water retention mechanism might be better than to use diuretic drugs. As mentioned in the chapter on hypertension, the water retention might come from three different mechanisms. The compound of ring-closed ANP to ring-opened ANP by the degradation of neutral endopeptidase (NEP) (Wilkins, et al., 1993; Seymour, et al., 1994) is one of the mechanisms. Another is the Ang(1-7) formed directly from either Ang I or angiotensinogen also by the cleavage action of the same enzyme NEP (proposed hypothetically). The water retention from Ang III by angiotensinase from the substrate Ang II could be automatically abolished in the presence of an ACE inhibitor. NEP inhibitors, such as SQ 28603 (Delaney et al., 1994), can stop the degradation by NEP activity to ring-opened ANP and Ang(1-7) formation. Simultaneously, both of the water retention mechanisms are abolished. Thus, the extra amount of water will no longer stay in the body. Mixed inhibitors of ACE and NEP may be very effective for low renin hypertensive treatment in patients. Unfortunately, SQ 28603 is not available yet as a drug on the market. Water pill (HCTZ) can be used as a substitute for SQ 28603.

The ACE active-site is well established. The binding knowledge of an inhibitor to NEP with the aid of a similar binding model of the ACE active-site is also quite well understood. Synthesizing a NEP inhibitor is not a problem. NEP and ACE inhibitors synthesized as one single compound for two different treatments may not be that easy. Compounds (called dual inhibitors) (Fig. 30), such as RB105, BMS 182657 and Omapatrilat (and others), have been already synthesized. Those inhibitors are indicated for the treatment of hypertension and congestive heart failure (Seymour et al., 1993; Tripodo et al., 1996 and 1998; Gonzalez, et al., 1996). Those dual inhibitors, theoretically, should be very effective for hypertension involving all levels of renin (low, moderate and high renin).

One thing worth mentioning is that in the late 70's, the original idea to design the NEP inhibitor was not for inhibiting the substrates of ANP, Ang I and angiotensinogen from the NEP cleavage activity. It was to design analgesic compounds for inhibiting the enkephalinase enzyme activity that degrades the substrate enkephalin which showed potent analgesic effects (Roemer, et al., 1977; Malfory, et al., 1978; Wilkins, et al., 1993) (Fig. 31). Enkephalinase was also referred to as NEP later. With the aid of the binding model of angiotensin-converting enzyme, the enkephalinase (NEP) inhibitor was obtained, such as thiorphan, SQ 28133 and then SQ 28603. NEP activity was inhibited for the substrate enkephalin in the presence of these inhibitors. However, a good indicator for analgesic effects in animal models could not be found at that time and it was not pursued further. Theoretically, if enkephalin is a true analgesic compound and present in the body, the analgesic effect will be presented. The analgesic effect of endorphin and enkephalin are well documented. The NEP inhibitor will stop the degradation of enkephalin by NEP activity. Analgesic effects will result from this inhibition. Dual inhibitor is a compound combining both the functions of ACE inhibition and NEP inhibition in one single compound. This kind of inhibitor may benefit all kinds of renin hypertension (high, moderate and low renin). Of course, NEP inhibition from this dual inhibitor plays a very important role in this treatment. As a result of this NEP inhibition by the dual inhibitor, the analgesic effect may be present along with hypertension and congested heart failure treatment. Thus, dual inhibitor may be of benefit for patients with pain.

Two different functional compounds synthesized in one single compound

For some patients who could not take an ACE inhibitor for anti-hypertensive treatment because of coughing, Ang II receptor antagonist was a very effective drug. The above mentioned dual inhibitor will have the same coughing effect for those patients because of ACE inhibition. The part of the structure for ACE inhibition in dual inhibitor could be substituted with a portion of the configuration of Ang II receptor antagonist. This new compound would not contribute ACE inhibition and the coughing effect would not occur. This proposed drug (dual function inhibitor, enzyme inhibitor and receptor blocker) could possibly be very effective and as good as dual inhibitor but without the occurrence of coughing. Not many scientists are aware of the possibility of this concept. Thus, no such compound has been synthesized.

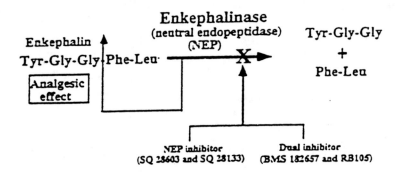

Fig. 31. Neutral endopeptidase activity with
substrate enkephalin

Final Conclusion and Comment

Hypertension is one of the most common diseases in human. The hard pulse was known 4000 years ago by Chinese emperor Huang-Ti. He commented that people who ate too much salt had hard pulse. The instrument for measuring blood pressure now used everyday by physicians, nurses and others was invented 100 years ago. Knowledge for understanding hypertension today is much clearer. The drug design for ACE inhibitors in hypertension is well established. Unanswered questions are awaiting answers in the near future. The human brain is the most important, vital tool to answer the questions and fix the problems. Any other tools including computers, biotechnology (including the concept of molecular biology and the gene) or high technology and others are used to help and enhance the function of the brain. The importance of the brain is not in any circumstance to be replaced by those tools. Thus, we need the external tools for aiding but not replacing the brain.

* * *

References

Bakhle, Y.S., 1972. Inhibition of converting enzyme by venom peptides. In Hyperyension. eds. J. Genest and E. Koiw, pp. 541-547. New York: Springer

Blair-West, J.R., Coghlan, J.P., Denton, D.A., Funder, J.W., Scoggins, B.A. and Wrighy, R.D. 1971. The effect of the heptapeptide (2-8) and hexapeptide (3-8) fragments of angiotensin II on aldosterone secretion. J Clin Endocrinol Metab 32:575-578

Boyd, G.W., Adamson, A.R., Fitz, A.E. and Peart, W.S. 1969. Radio-immunoassay determination of plasma-renin activity. Lancet 7588:213-218

Byers, L.D. and Wolfenden, R. 1972. A potent reversible inhibitor of carboxypeptidase A. J Biol Chem 247:606-608

Byers, L.D. and Wolfenden, R. 1973. Binding of the biproduct analog benzylsuccinic by carboxypeptidase A. Biochemistry 12:2070-2078

Cambell, W.B., Brooks, S.N. and Pettinger, W.A. 1974. Angiotensin II and angiotensin III-induced aldosterone release in vivo in the rat. Science 125:886-887

Chan, W.K., Chan, T.Y.K., Luk, W.K., Leung, V.K.S., Li, T.H. and Critchley, J.A.J.H. 1993. A high incidence of cough in chinese subjects treated with angiotensin-converting enzyme inhibitors. Eur J Clin Pharmacol 44:299-300

Cheung, H.S. and Cushman, D.W. 1973a. Inhibition of homogeneous angiotensin-converting enzyme of rabbit lung by synthetic venom peptides of Bothrops jararaca. Biochem Biophys Acta 293:451-463

Cheung, H.S. and Cushman, D.W. 1973b. Mechanism of inhibition of angiotensin-converting enzyme by Venom peptides. Federation Proc 32:765

Cheung, H.S., Wang, F.L., Ondetti, M.A., Sabo, E.F. and Cushman, D.W. 1980. Binding of peptide substrates and inhibitors of angiotensin-converting enzyme. Importance of the COOH terminal dipeptide sequence. J Biol Chem 255:401-407

Cheung, H.S. 1996. A historical account of rational design of captopril, the first angiotensin-converting enzyme inhibitor in treatment of hyper-tension. Bio/Pharma Quarterly 2:1-5

Cheung, H.S. 1997. The concept for designing tripeptide angiotensin-converting enzyme inhibitor as drug in treatment of hypertension. Bio/Pharma Quarterly 3:1-2

Chiu, A.T., Carini, D.J., Johnson, A.L., McCall, D.E., Price, W.A., Thoolen, M.J.M.C., Wong, P.C., Taber, R.I. and Timmermans. P.B.M.W.M. 1988. Non-peptide angiotensin II receptor antagonists. II. Pharmacology of S-8308. Eur J Pharmacol 157:13-21

Chiu, A.T., McCall, D.E., Price, W.A., Wong, P.C., Carini, D.J., Duncia, J.V., Wexler, R.R., Yoo, S.E., Johnson, A.L. and Timmermans, P.B.M.W.M. 1990. Nonpeptide angiotensin II receptor antagonist. VII. cellular and biochemical pharmacology of DuP 753, an orally active antihypertensive agent. J Pharmacol Exp Ther 252:711-718

Cushman, D.W. and Cheung, H.S. 1971. Spectrophotometric essay and properties of the angiotensin-converting enzyme of rabbit lung, Biochem Pharmacol 20:1637-1648

Cushman, D.W. and Cheung, H.S. 1972. Studies in vitro of angiotensin-converting enzyme of lung and other tissues. In Hypertwnsion. eds. J. Genest and E. Koiw, pp.532-541, New York: Springer

Cushman, D.W., Plušcec, J., Williams, N.J., Weaver, E.R., Sabo, E.F., Kocy, O., Cheung, H.S. and Ondetti, M.A. 1973. Inhibition of angiotensin-converting enzyme by analogs of peptides from Bothrops jararaca venom. Experientia 29:1032-1035

Cushman, D.W., Cheung, H.S., Sabo, E.F. and Ondetti, M.A. 1977. Design of potent competitive inhibitors of angiotensin-converting enzyme. Carboxyalkanoyl and mercaptoalkanoyl amino acids. Biochemistry 16:5484-5491

Cushman, D.W., Cheung, H.S., Sabo, E.F. and Ondetti, M.A. 1978. Design of new antihypertensive drugs: potent and specific inhibitors of angiotensin-converting enzyme. Prog Cardiovasc Dis 21:176-182

Cushman, D.W., Cheung, H.S., Sabo, E.F. and Ondetti, M.A. 1979. Development of specific inhibitors of angiotensin I converting enzyme (kininase II) Fed Proc 38:2778-2782

Cushman, D.W. and Ondetti, M.A. 1980. Inhibition of angiotensin-converting enzyme for treatment of hypertension. Biochem Pharmacol 29:1871-1877

Cushman, D.W., Cheung, H.S., Sabo, E.F. Ondetti, M.A. 1981. Angiotensin converting enzyme inhibitors: evolution of a new class of antihypertension drugs. In Angiotensin Converting Enzyme Inhibitors, Mechanisms of Action and Clinical Implications, ed. Z.P. Horovitz, pp. 3-25. Maryland: Urban & Schwarzenberg

Delaney, G.N., Barrish, J.C., Neubeck, R., Natarajan, S., Cohen, M., Rovnyak, G.C., Huber, G., Murugesan, N., Girotra, R., Sieber-McMaster, E., Robl, J.A., Asaad, M.M., Cheung, H.S., Bird, J.E., Waldron, T., and Petrillo, E.W. 1994. Mercaptoacyl dipeptides as dual inhibitors of angiotensin-converting enzyne and neutral endopeptidase. preliminary structure-activity studies. Bioorg & Medicinal Chem Letters 4:1783-1788

Dorer, F.E., Skeggs, L.T., Hahn, J.R., Lentz, K.E. and Levine, M. 1970. Angiotensin-converting enzyme: method of assay and partial purification Anal. Biochem 33:102-113

Engel, S.L., Schaeffer, T.R., Gold, B.I. and Rubin, B. 1972. Inhibition of pressor effects of angiotensin I and augmentation of depressor effect of bradykinin by synthetic peptides. Proc Soc Exp Biol Med 140:240-244

Erdös, E.G. 1977. The angiotensin I converting enzyme. Federation Proc 36:1760-1765

Ferreira, S.H., Greene, L.J., Alabaster, V.A., Bakhle, Y.S. and Vane, J.R. 1970a. Activity of various fractions of bradykinin potentiating factor against angiotensin I converting enzyme. Nature 225:379-380

Ferreira, S.H., Bartelt, D.C. and Greene, L.J. 1970b Isolation of brady-kinin potentiating peptides from Bothrops jararaca venom. Biochemistry 9:2583-2593

Fletcher, A.E., Palmer, A.J. and Bulpitt, C.J. 1994. Cough with angiotensin converting enzyme inhibitors: how much of a problem?.
J Hypertens 12:S43-S47

Gonzalez, W.,Beslot, F., Laboulandine, I., Fourne-Zaluski, M.C., Roques, B.P. and Michel, J.B. 1996. Inhibition of both angiotensin-converting enzyme and neutral endopeptidase by S21402 (Rb105) in rats with experimental myocardial infraction. J Pharmacol Exp Ther 278:573-581

Goodfriend, J.L. and Peach, M. J. 1975. Angiotensin III: (des-aspartic acid)-angiotensin II. evidence and speculation for its role as an important agonist in the renin-angiotensin system. Circ Res 36-37 (Suppl. 1):38-48

Greene, L.J., Camargo, A.C.M., Krieger, E.M., Stewart, J.M. and Ferreira, S.H. 1972. Inhibition of the conversion of angiotensin I to II and potentiation of bradykinin by small peptidase present in Bothrops jararaca venom. Circ Res 30:II-62-II-71

Hartsuck, J.A., and Lipscomb, W.N. 1971 Carboxypeptidase A. In The Enzyme, Vol. 3. Ed. P.D. Boyer, pp.1-56. : ..w York: Academic Press

Helmer, O.M. 1957. Difference between two forms of angiotensin by means of spirally cut strips of rabbit aorta. Am J Physiol 188:571-577

Hoffmann, K. and Bergmann, M.. 1946. The specificity of carboxy-peptidase. J Biol Chem 134:225-235

Hollemans, H.J.G., Van Der Meer, J. and Kloosterziel, W. 1969. Identification of the incubation product of Boucher's renin activity assay, by means of radioimmunoassays for angiotensin I and angiotensin II , and a converting enzyme preparation from lung tissue. Clin Chim Acta 23:7-15

Lacourciere, Y., Lefebvre, J., Nakhle, G., Faison, E.P., Snavely, D.B. and Nelson, E.B. 1994. Association between cough and angiotensin converting enzyme inhibitors versus angiotensin II antagonists: the design of a prospective, controlled study. J Hypertens 12:S49-S53

Lentz, K.E., Skeggs, L.T., Jr., Wood,K.R., Kahn, J.R., and Shumway, N.P. 1956. The amino acid composition of Hypertensin II and its biochemical relationship to hypertensin I. J Exp Med 104:183-191

Liorens, C., Gacel, G., Swerts, J.P., Perdrisot, R., Fournie-Zaluski, M.C., Schwartz, J.C., and Roques, B.P. 1980. Rational design of enkephalinase inhibitors: substrate specificity of enkephalinase studied from inhibitory potency of various dipeptides. Biochem Biophys Res Comm. 96:1710-1716

Malfory, B., Swerts, J.P., Guyon, A., Roques, B.P. and Schwartz, J.C. 1978. High-affinity enkephalin-degrading peptidase in brain is increased after morphine. Nature 276:523-526

O'Brien, E. and Fitzgerald, D. 1994. The history of blood pressure measurement. J Human Hypertension 8:73-84

Ondetti M.A., Williams, N.J., Sabo, E.F., Plušček, J., Weaver, E.R. and Kocy, O. 1971. Angiotensin-converting enzyme inhibitors from the venom of Bothrops jararaca, elucidation of structure and synthesis. Biochemistry 10:4033-4039

Ondetti, M.A., Rubin, B. and Cushman, D.W. 1977. Design of Specific inhibitors of angiotensin-converting enzyme: A new Class of orally active antihypertensive agents. Science 196:441-444

Page, L.B., Haber, E., Kimura, A.Y. and Purnode A. 1969. Studies with the radioimmunoassay for angiotensin II and its application to measurement of renin activity. J Clin Endor Metab 29:200-206

Roemer, D., Buescher, H.H., Hill, R.C., Pless, J., Bauer, W., Cardinaux, F., Closse, A., Hauser, D. and Huggenin, R. 1977. A synthetic enkephalin analogue with proloned parenteral and oral analgesic activity. Nature 268:547-549

Roques, B.P., Fournic-Zaluski, M. C., Soroca, E., Lecomte, J.M., Malfroy, B and Liorens, C. 1980. The enkephalinase inhibitor thiorphan show antinociceptive activity in mice. Nature 288:286-288

Rubin, B. and Antonaccio. M.J. 1980. Captopril. In Pharmacology of Antihypertensive Drugs. ed. A. Scriabine, pp.21-42. New York: Raven Press

Ryan, J.W., Roblero, J and Stewart, J.M. 1968. Inactivation of brady-kinin in the pulmonary circulation. Biochem J 110:795-797

Santos, R.A.S. and Campagnole-Santos M.J. 1994. Central and peripheral actions of angiotensin-(1-7). Brazllian J MED Biol Res 27:1033-1047

Seymour, A.A., Asaad, M., Lanoce, V.M., Fennel, S.A., Cheung, H.S. and Rogers, L.W. 1993. Inhibition of neutral endopeptidase 3.4.24.11 in concious dogs with pacing induced heart failure. Cardiovas Res 27:1015-1023

Seymour, A.A., Sheldon, J.H., Smith, L.P., Asaad, M. and Rogers, L. 1994. Potentiation of the renal responses to bradykinin by inhibition of neutral endopeptidase 3.4.24.11 and angiotensin-converting enzyme in anesthetized dogs. J Pharmacol Exp Ther 269:263-270

Shevchenko, Y.L. and Tsithk, J.E. 1996. 90th anniversary of the development by Nicolai S. Korotkoff of the auscultatory method of measuring blood pressure. Circulation 94:116-118

Skeggs, L.T., Marsh, W.H., Kahn, J.R. and Shumway, N.P. 1954. The existence of two forms of hypertension. J Exp Med 99:275-282

Skeggs, L.T., Kahn, J.R., and Shumway, N.P. 1956. The preparation and function of the hypertension-converting enzyme. J Exp Med 103:295-299

Stewart, J.M., Ferreira, S.H. and Greene, L.J. 1971. Bradykinin-potentiating peptide PCA-Lys-Trp-Ala-Pro. An inhibitor of the pulmonary inactivation of bradykinin and conversion of angiotensin I to II. Biochem Pharmacol 20:1557-1567

Tripodo, N.C., Robl, J.A., Asaad, M.M., Eileen Bird, J, Panchal, B.C., Schaeffer, T.R., Fox, M., Giancarli, M.R. and Cheung, H.S. 1996. Cardiovascular effects of the novel dual inhibitor of neutral endopeptidase and angiotensin-converting enzyme BMS-182657. J Pharmaco Exp Therap 275:745-752

Tripodo, N.C., Robl, J.A., Asaad, M.M., Fox, M., Panchal, B.C., and Schaeffer, T.R. 1998. Effects of Omapatrilat in low, normal and high rennin experimental hypertension. Am. J. Hypertens 11:363-372

Wilkins, M.R. Unwin, R.J. and Kenny, A.J. 1993. Endopeptidase-24.11 and its inhibitors: potential therapeutic agents for edematous disorders and hypertension. Kidney international. 43:273-285

Wong, P.C., Price, W.A., Chiu, A.T., Thoolen, M.J.M.C., Duncia, J.V., Johnson, A.L., and Timmermans, P.B.M.W.M. 1989. Nonpeptide angiotensin II receptor antagonist. IV. EXP6155 and Exp6803. Hypertension 13: 489-497

Yang, H.Y.T., Erdös, E.G. and Levin, Y. 1970. A dipeptidyl carboxypeptidase that converts angiotensin I and inactivates bradykinin. Biochem Biophys Acta 214:374-376

* Medications were prescribed and blood pressure was verified by
  Dr. Samuel Friedman.

Abbreviations

AA	Amino acid
ABS	Auxiliary binding site
ACE	Angiotensin-converting enzyme
AI	Angiotensin I
Ang I	Angiotensin I
Ang(1-10)	Angiotensin I
AII	Angiotensin II
Ang II	Angiotensin II
Ang(1-8)	Angiotensin II
Ang III	Angiotensin III
ANF	Atrial natriuretic factor
ANP	Atrial natriuretic peptide
CPase A	Carboxypeptidase A
EBCS	Essential binding and cleavage site
HCTZ	Hydrochlorothiazide
HHL	Hippuryl-Histidyl-Leucine
Hipp	Hippuryl or hippuric acid
HL	Histidyl-leucine
I_{50}	The concentration of inhibitor used to induce 50 % enzyme blockade (50 % enzyme activity)
mm	Millimeter
mM	Millimolar
mU	Milliunit
NEP	Neutral endopeptidase
N	Normal
nm	Nanometer
PRA	Plasma renin activity
Pyr (<glu)	Pyroglutamic acid
µg	Microgram

Index